How to Use This Book

Once upon a Medical/Surgical ward in a hospital near you, a Registered Nurse precepted countless nursing students and noticed a common problem throughout entire cohorts of nearby programs.

Intelligent, book-smart students seemed to lack an understanding of how all of the concepts they had learned fit together. Each piece of information taught in nursing school is an important piece of a puzzle.

Concept maps are one of the best ways to study how information fits together. But concept maps are time-consuming to create and fill with information… right?

Introducing **Lena Empyema's Master Mapper series**. You've got the Pharmacology Master Mapper in your hands. This book is a color-coordinated workbook of concept map templates to assist in studying large amounts of information and memorizing the most pertinent facts and figures.

Ideally, use this workbook either before or after class to fill out information in every box. Pharmacology is a beast. "I thought I was done with chemistry when I finished my pre-requisites!" Lena gets it. It's a rough class, and there's more information on the exams than you'll ever be able to memorize, right? Not if you streamline your studying and focus on the data that makes each drug *unique*, different from the rest.

Filling out concept maps for the drugs being covered in lecture *before* you attend class allows you to highlight the information that your professors emphasize during class, which could help you during your next exam.

Alternatively, filling out the concept maps *after* class facilitates a thorough review of each drug before the exam, which can be equally beneficial in terms of memorizing information.

Because each type of information (i.e., mechanisms of action, side effects, listing other drugs in the same class…) is present in the same place on each page, this workbook streamlines the process of flipping through pages of information before an exam to easily pick out the *unique* data specific to a certain disease.

To expand on that concept, as examples, there are many drugs that result in weight gain or nausea. But which drugs cause hyperactivity? Which ones cause the body to retain potassium?

You got this.

Exam dates sneak up on the best of us.

Make life easier for yourself.

Fill out the table of contents on Page 3 as you go for ease of looking up the maps you worked so hard to create. Utilize the blank pages opposite each map for taking additional notes, or capturing concepts that don't easily fit into the colored templates.

<u>Pro tip,</u> from someone who's been through it: invest in multi-colored pens and highlighters. Use one color for notes taken during independent study and another color of ink for information presented in class. Then have a highlighter to mark the content that was emphasized in class so you know where to focus for the exam.

Pharmacology classes are no easy feat. Then again, you are not just an average nursing student. You have the passion, intelligence, and commitment to conquer nursing school. Let **The Pharmacology Master Mapper Workbook** help you in your journey.

Think positively, and visualize your success as you study to help maintain your confidence during exams.

Lena hopes you secure an A+.

~Lena Empyema

TABLE OF CONTENTS

4.	37.	68.
5.	38.	69.
6.	39.	70.
7.	40.	71.
8.	41.	72.
9.	42.	73.
10.	43.	74.
11.	44.	75.
12.	45.	76.
13.	46.	77.
14.	47.	78.
15.	48.	79.
16.	49.	80.
17.	50.	81.
18.	51.	82.
20.	52.	83.
21.	53.	84.
22.	54.	85.
23.	55.	86.
24.	56.	87.
25.	57.	88.
26.	58.	89.
27.	59.	90.
28.	60.	91.
29.	61.	92.
30.	62.	93.
31.	63.	94.
32.	64.	95.
33.	65.	96.
34.	66.	97.
35.	67.	98.
36.	68.	99.

Study. Dominate. Repeat.

Date: Class: This content will appear on Exam #:

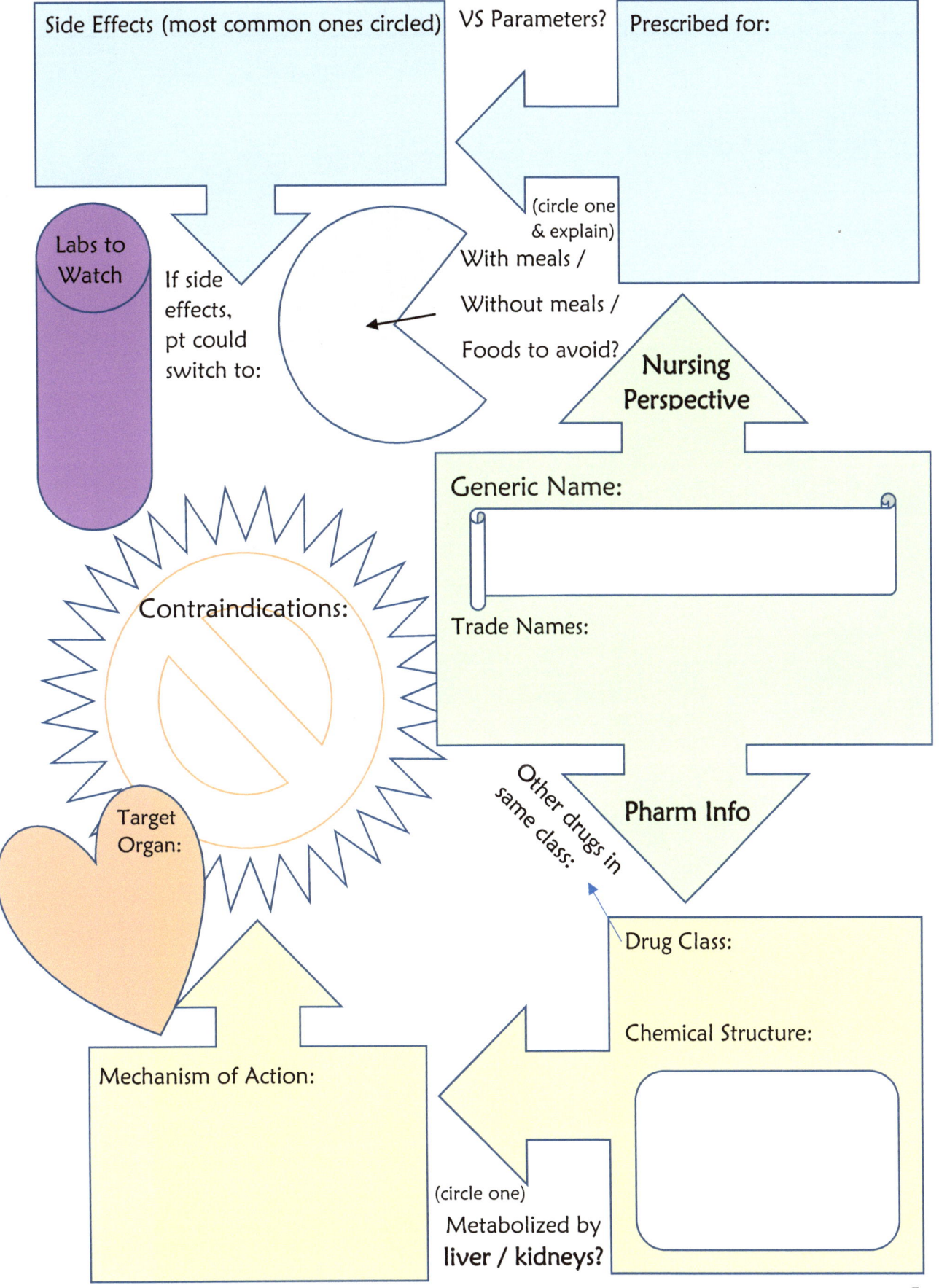

Date: Class: This content will appear on Exam #:

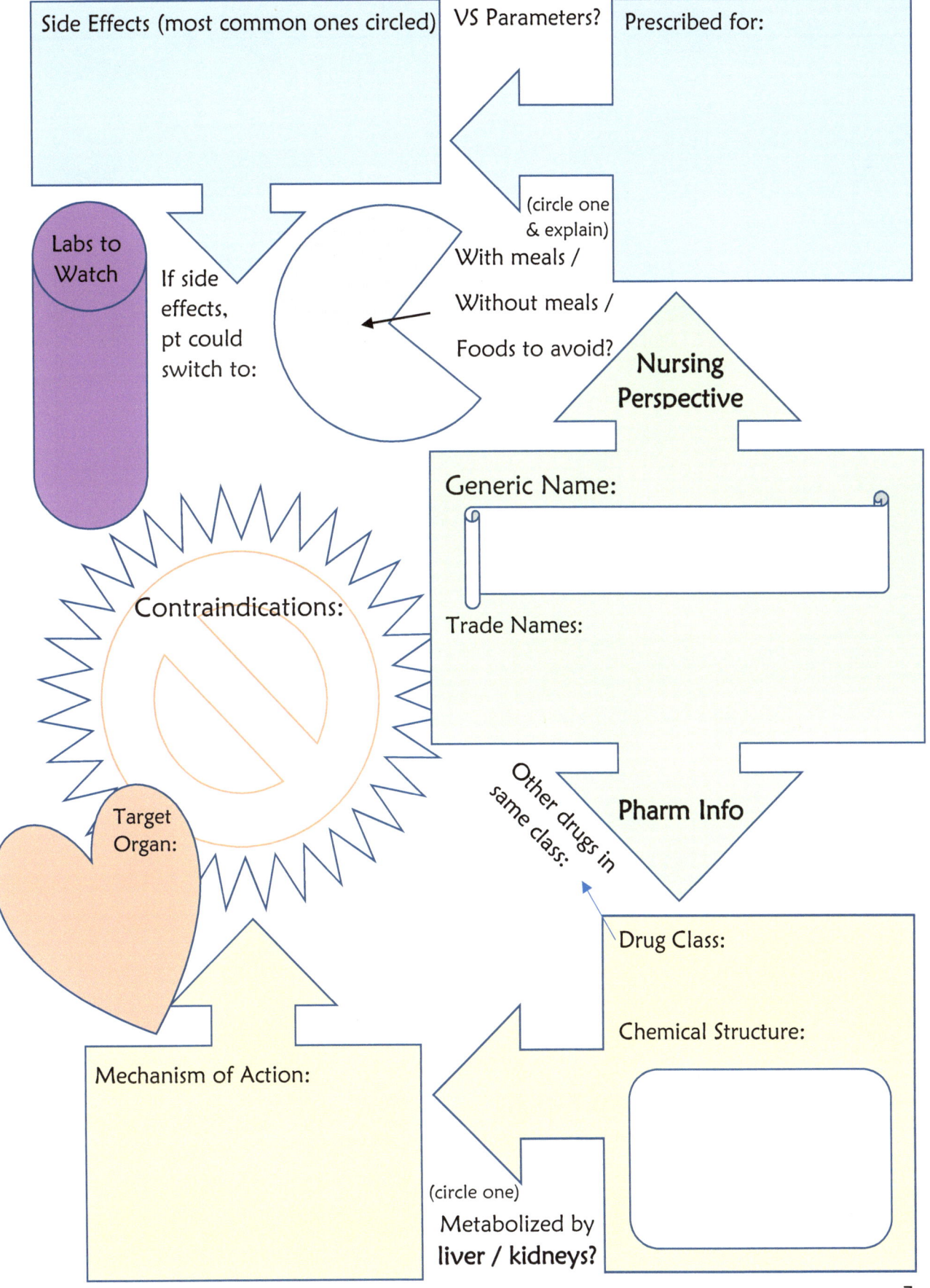

Date: Class: This content will appear on Exam #:

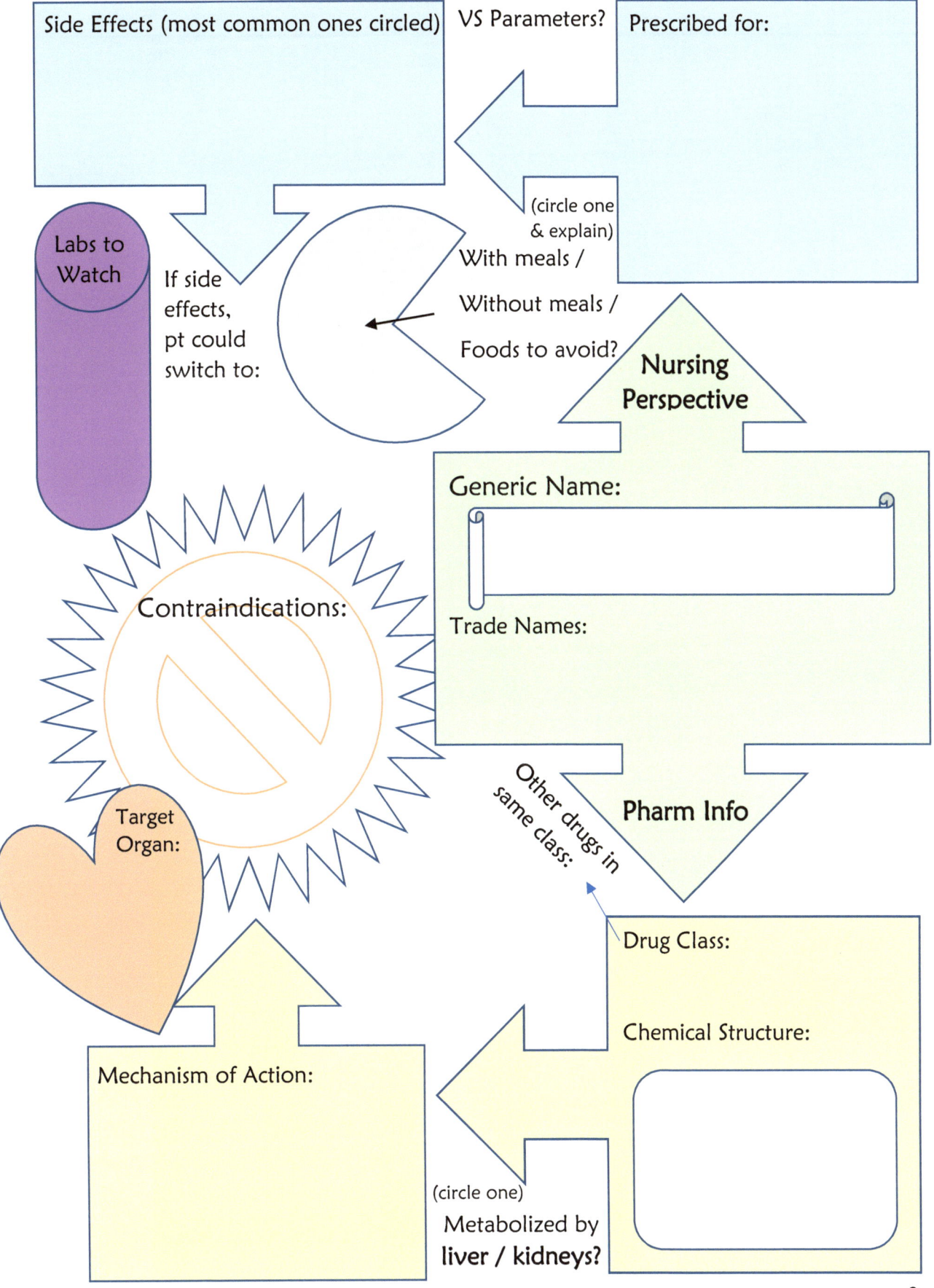

Date: Class: This content will appear on Exam #:

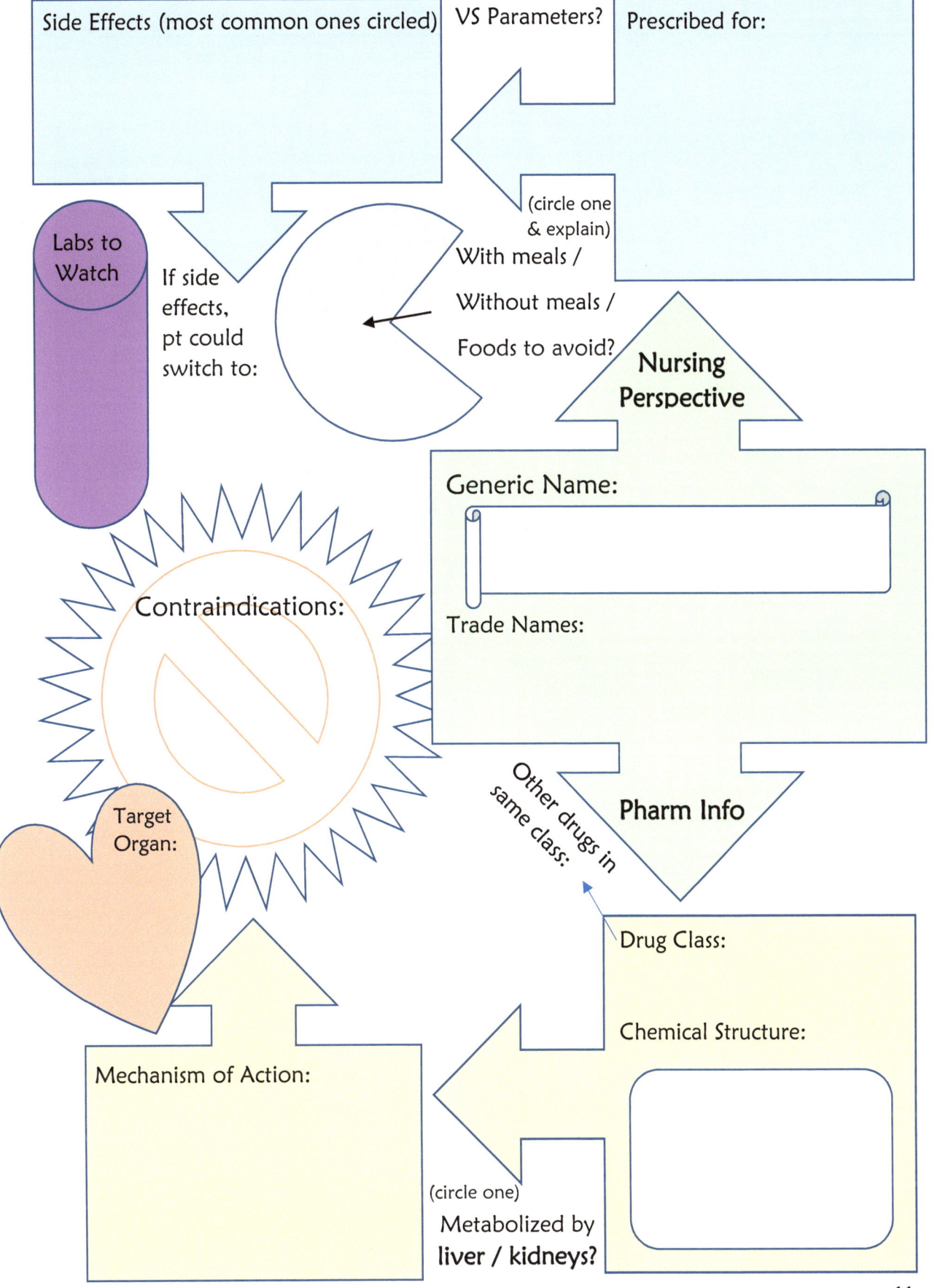

Date: Class: This content will appear on Exam #:

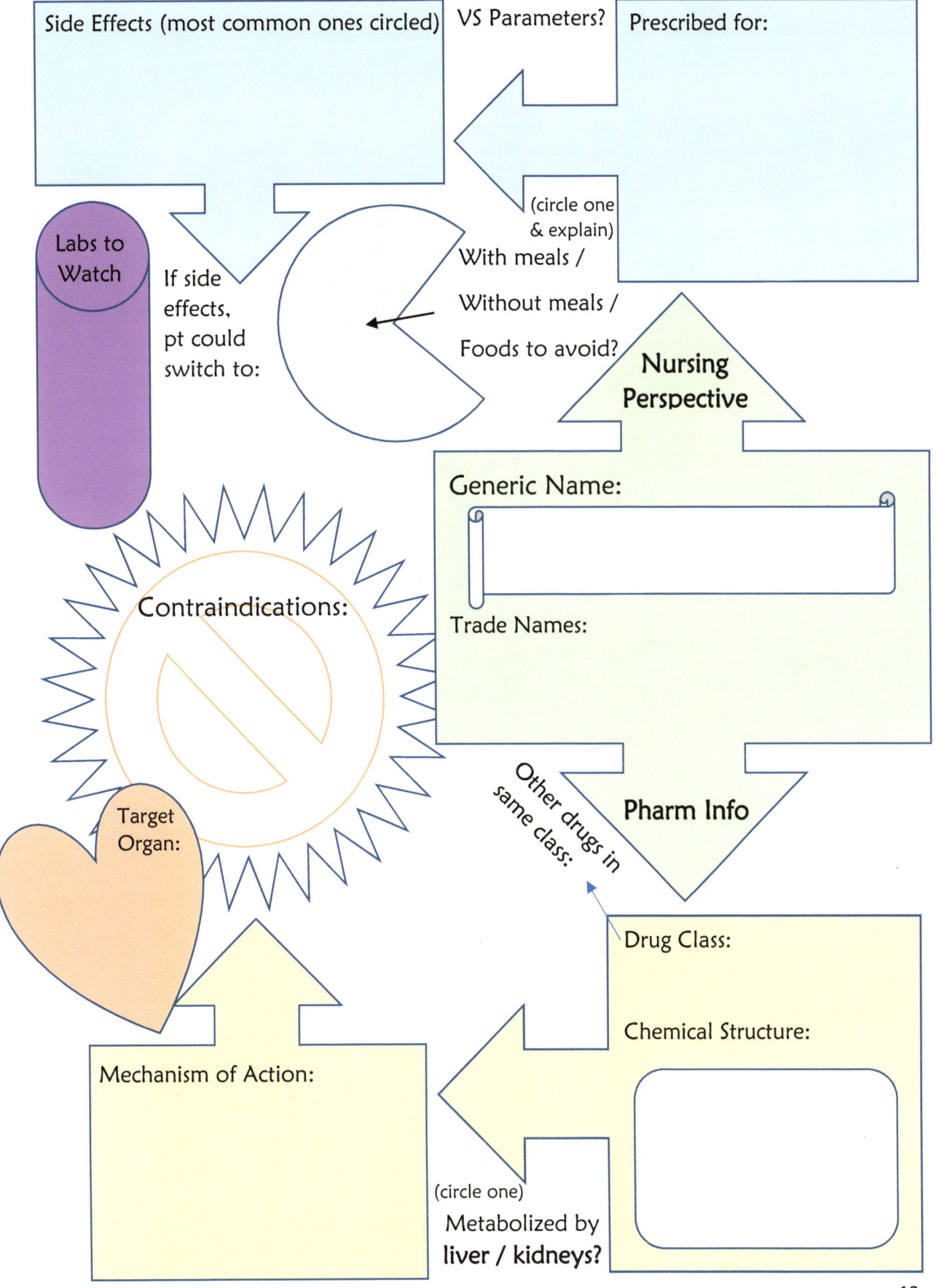

Date:	Class:	This content will appear on Exam #:

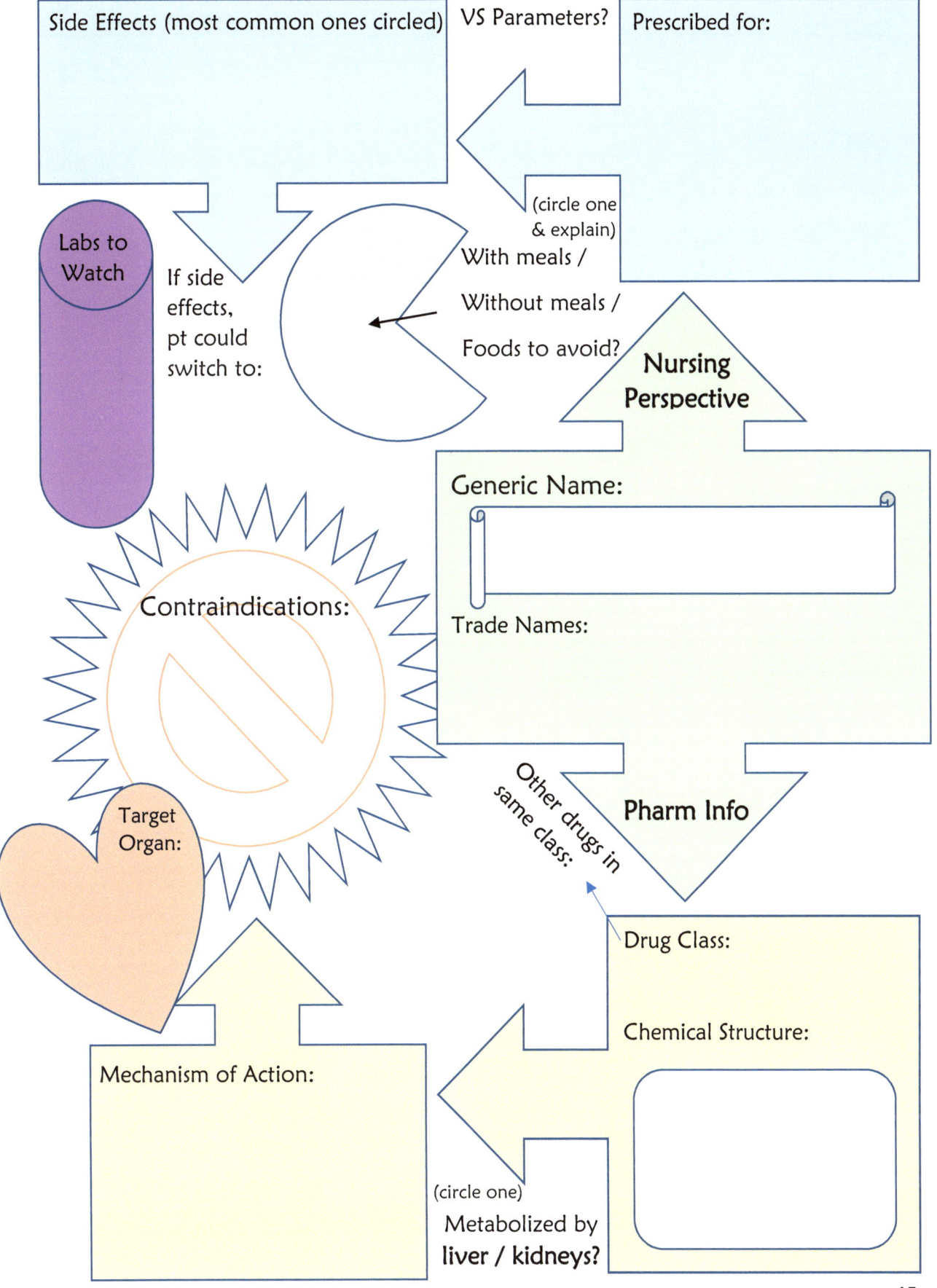

Date: Class: This content will appear on Exam #:

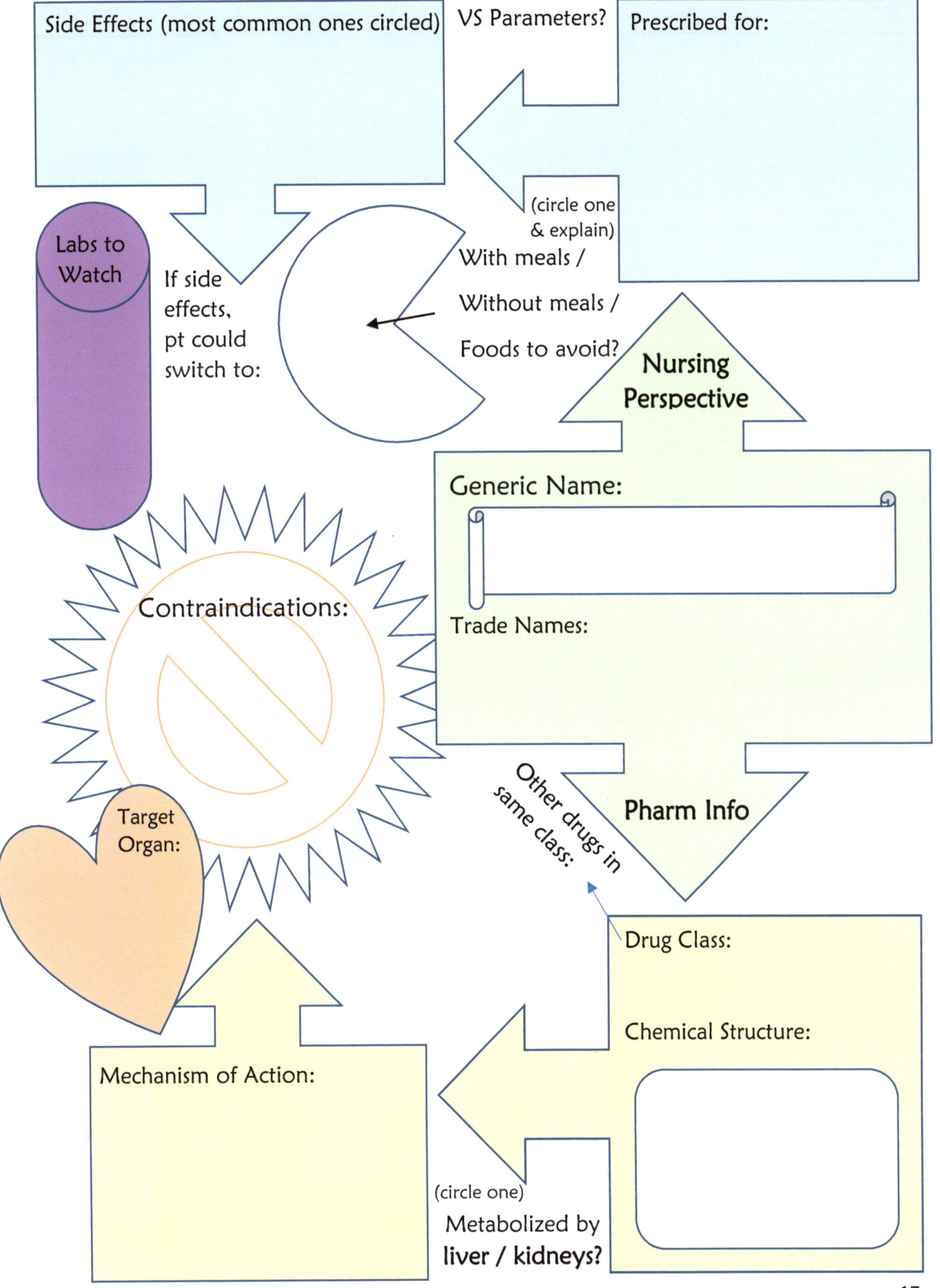

Date:	Class:	This content will appear on Exam #:

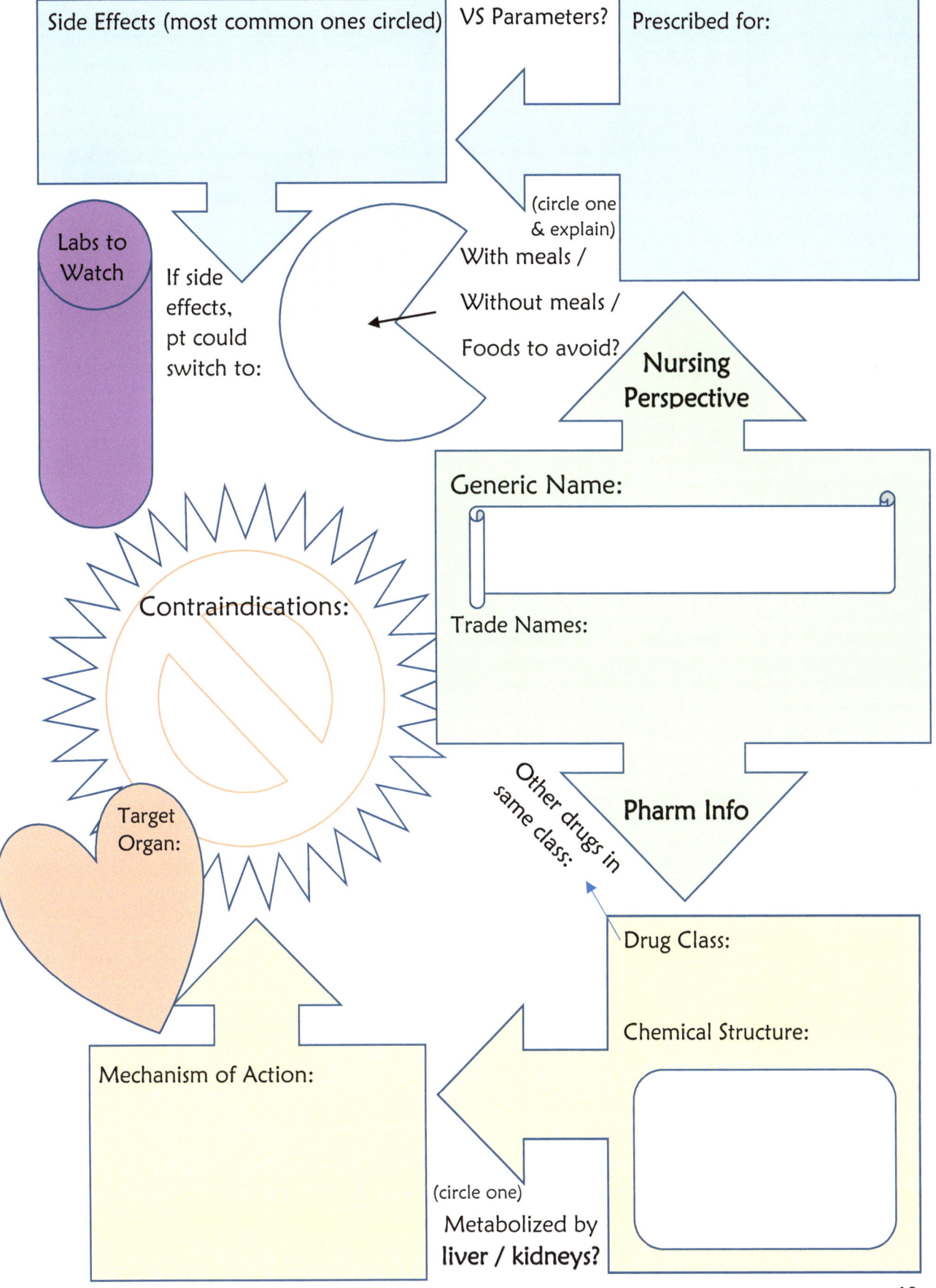

Date: Class: This content will appear on Exam #:

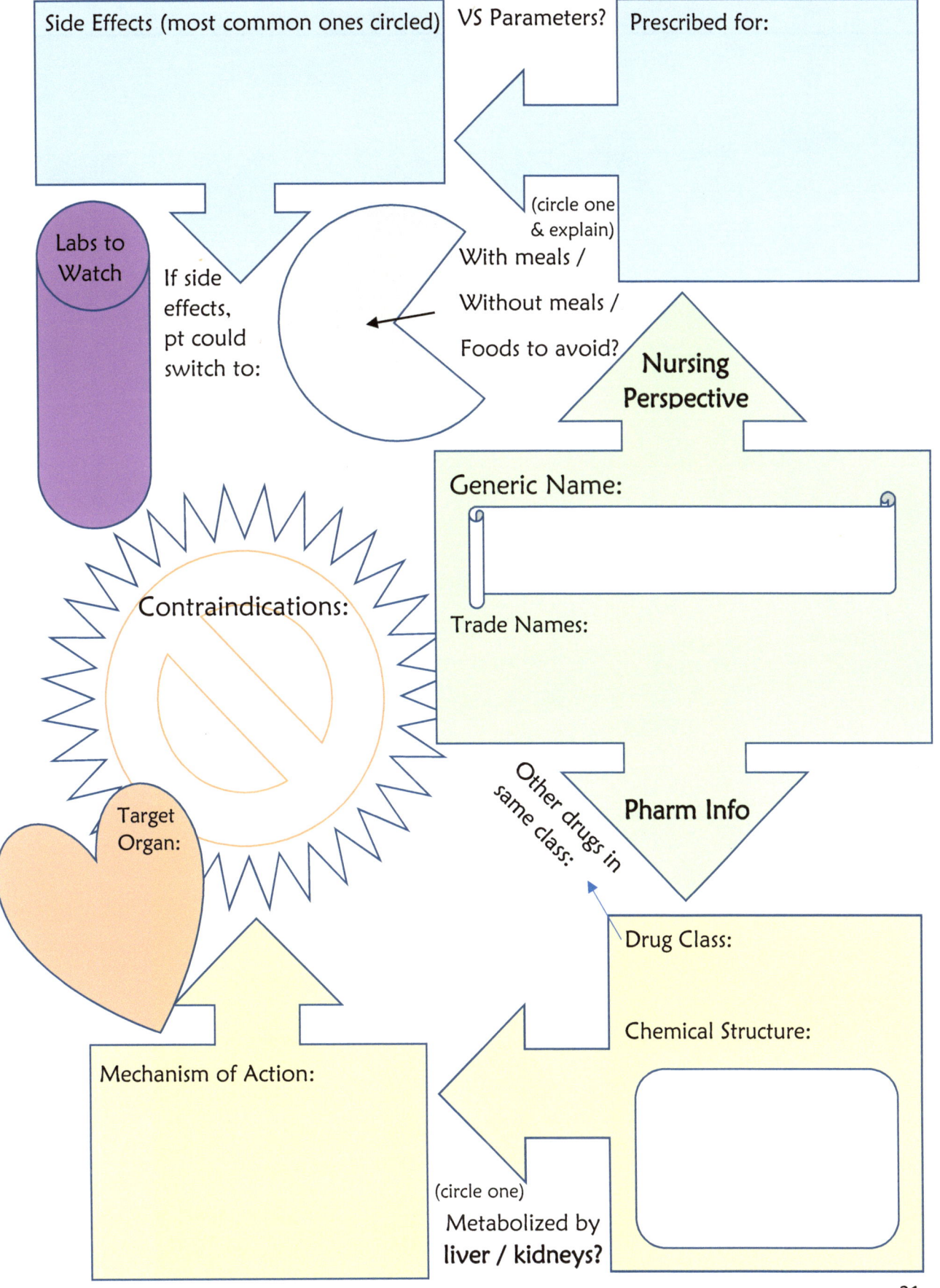

Date:　　　　　Class:　　　　　　　　This content will appear on Exam #:

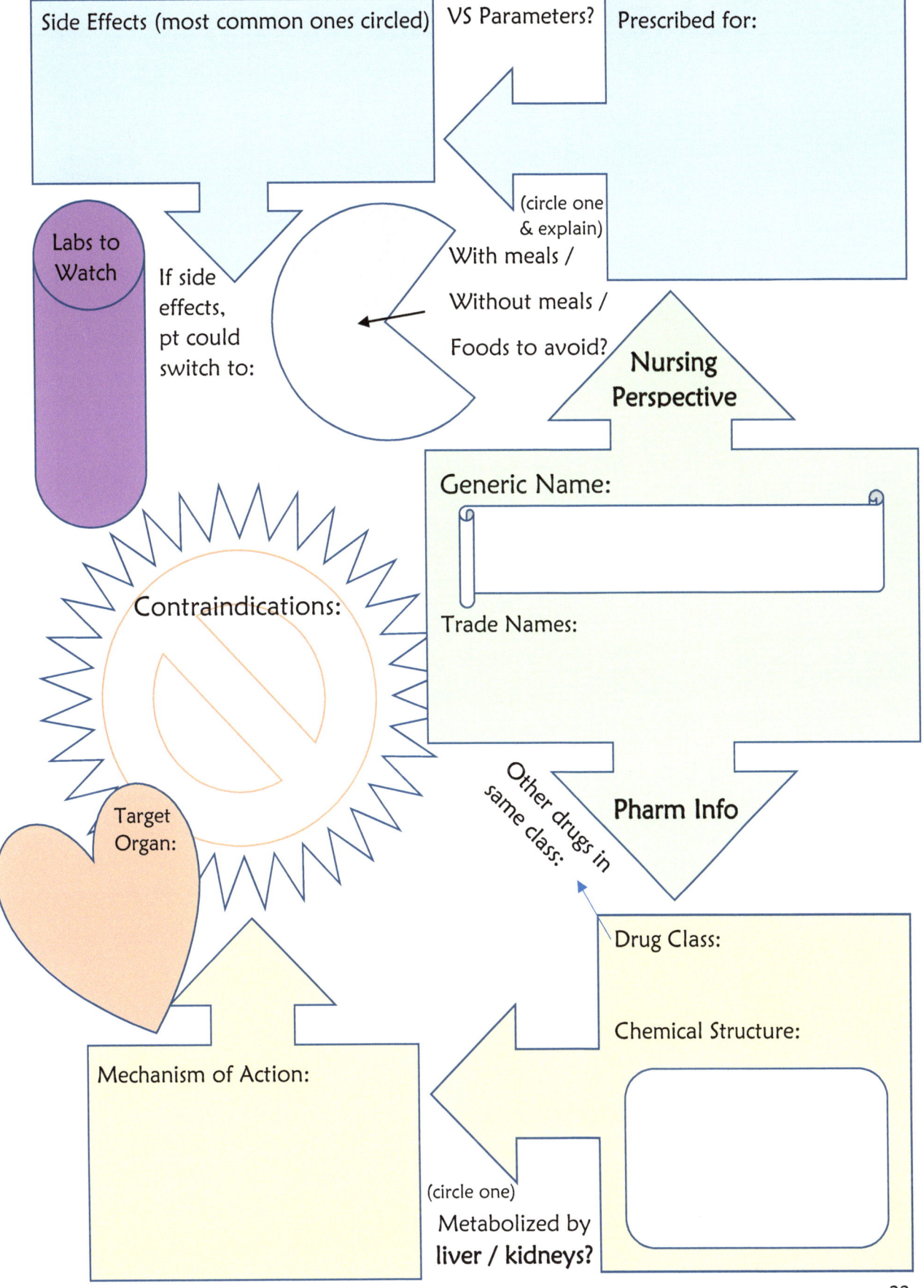

Date: Class: This content will appear on Exam #:

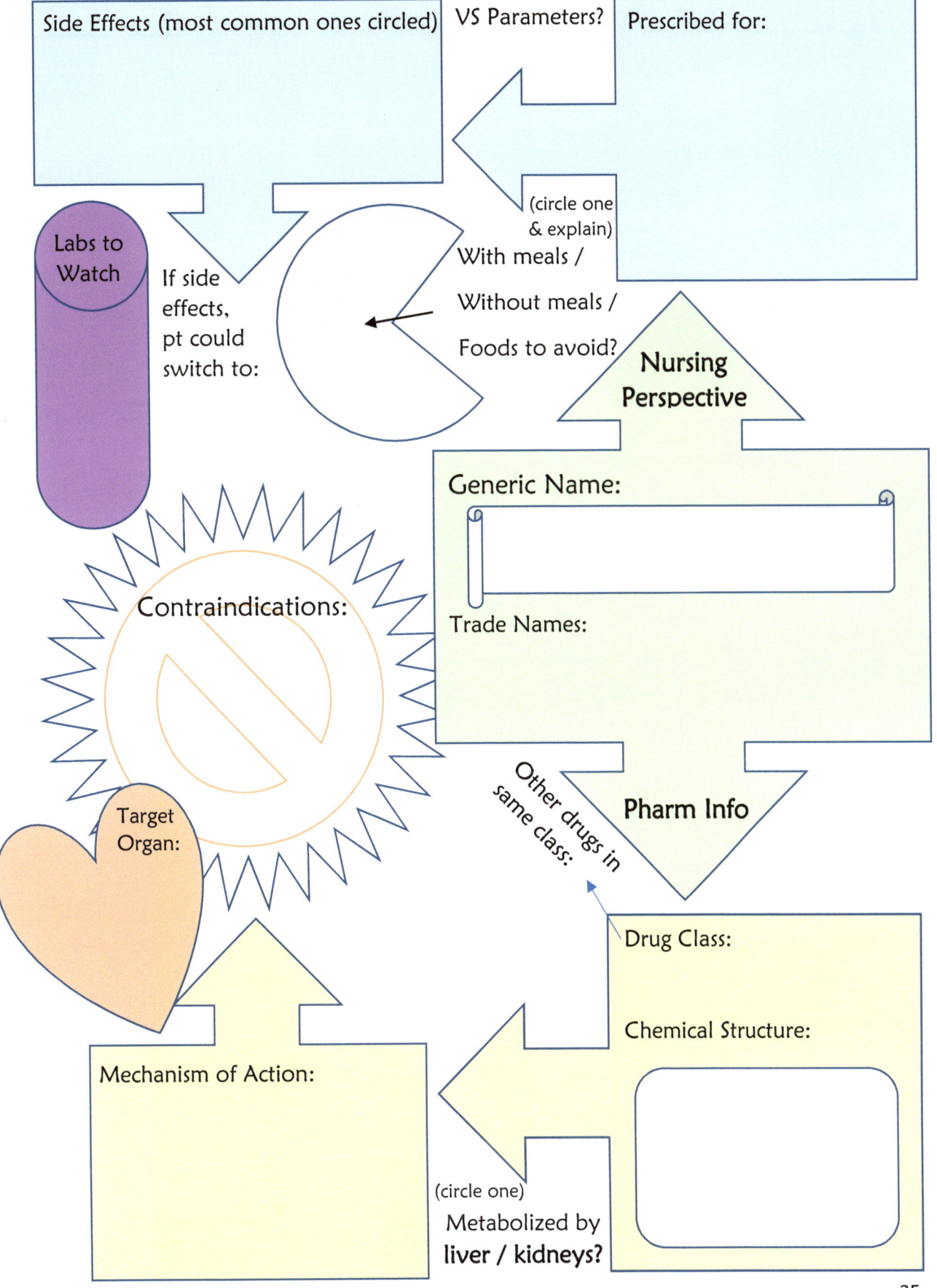

Date: Class: This content will appear on Exam #:

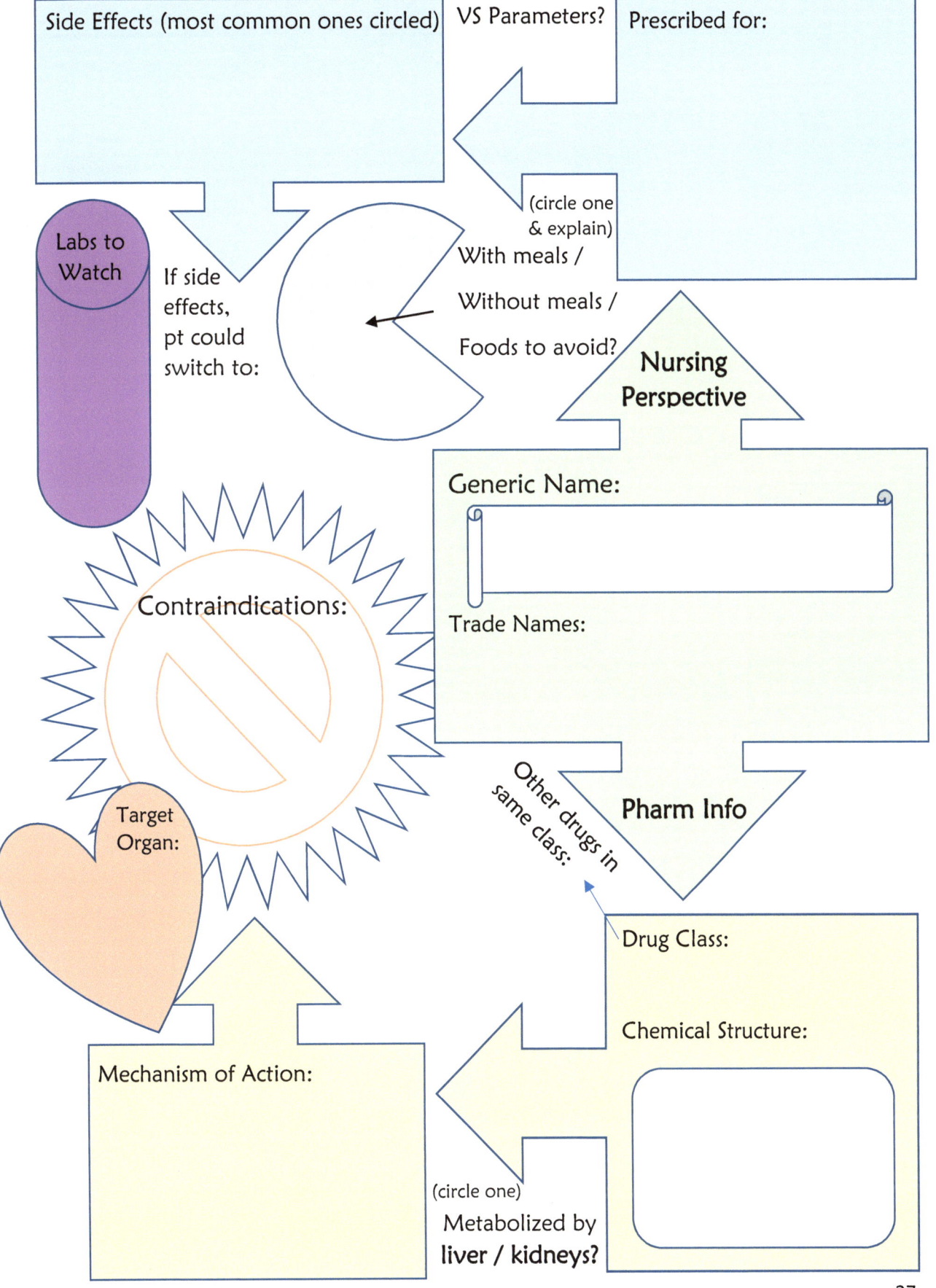

Date: Class: This content will appear on Exam #:

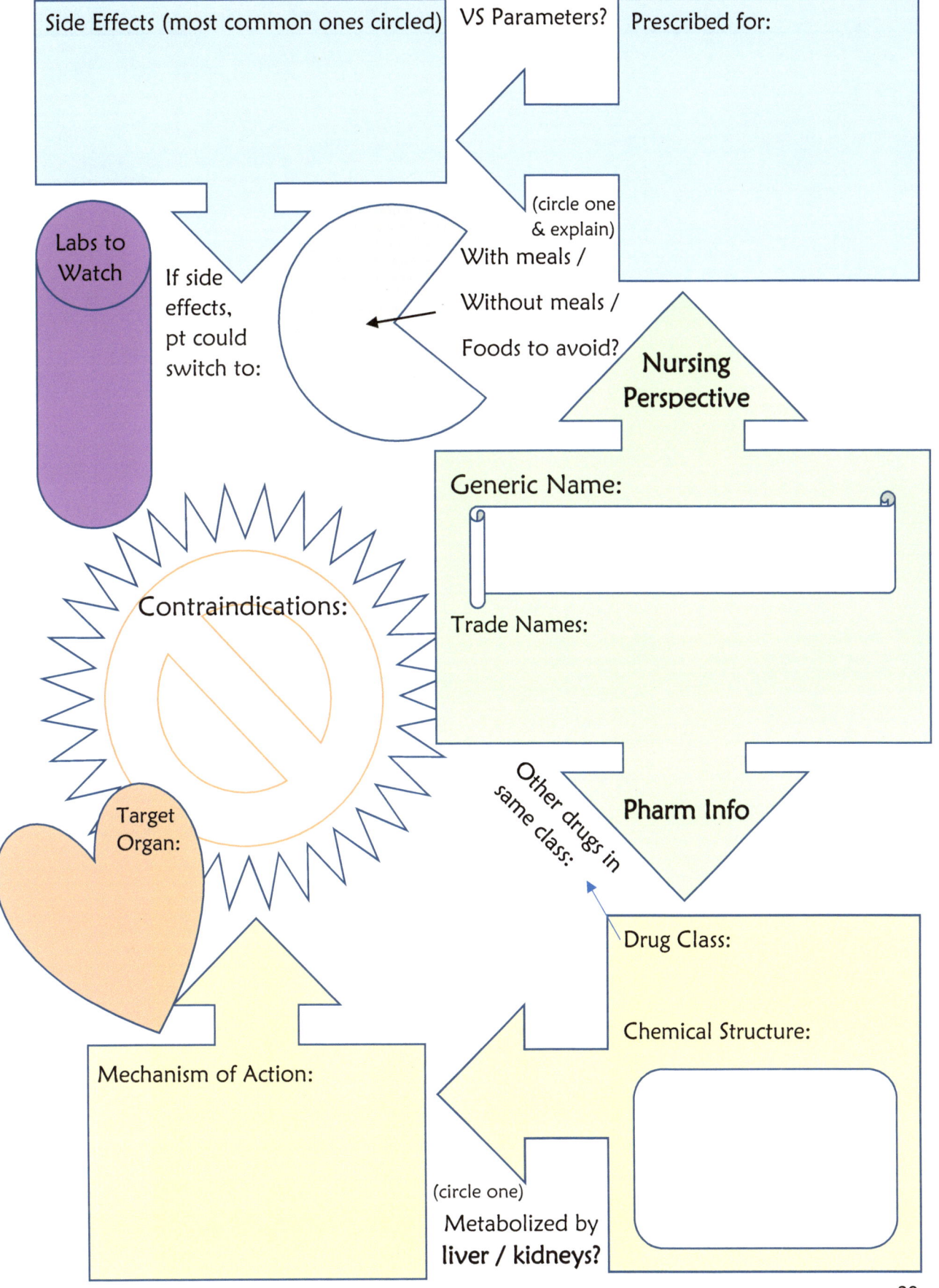

Date: Class: This content will appear on Exam #:

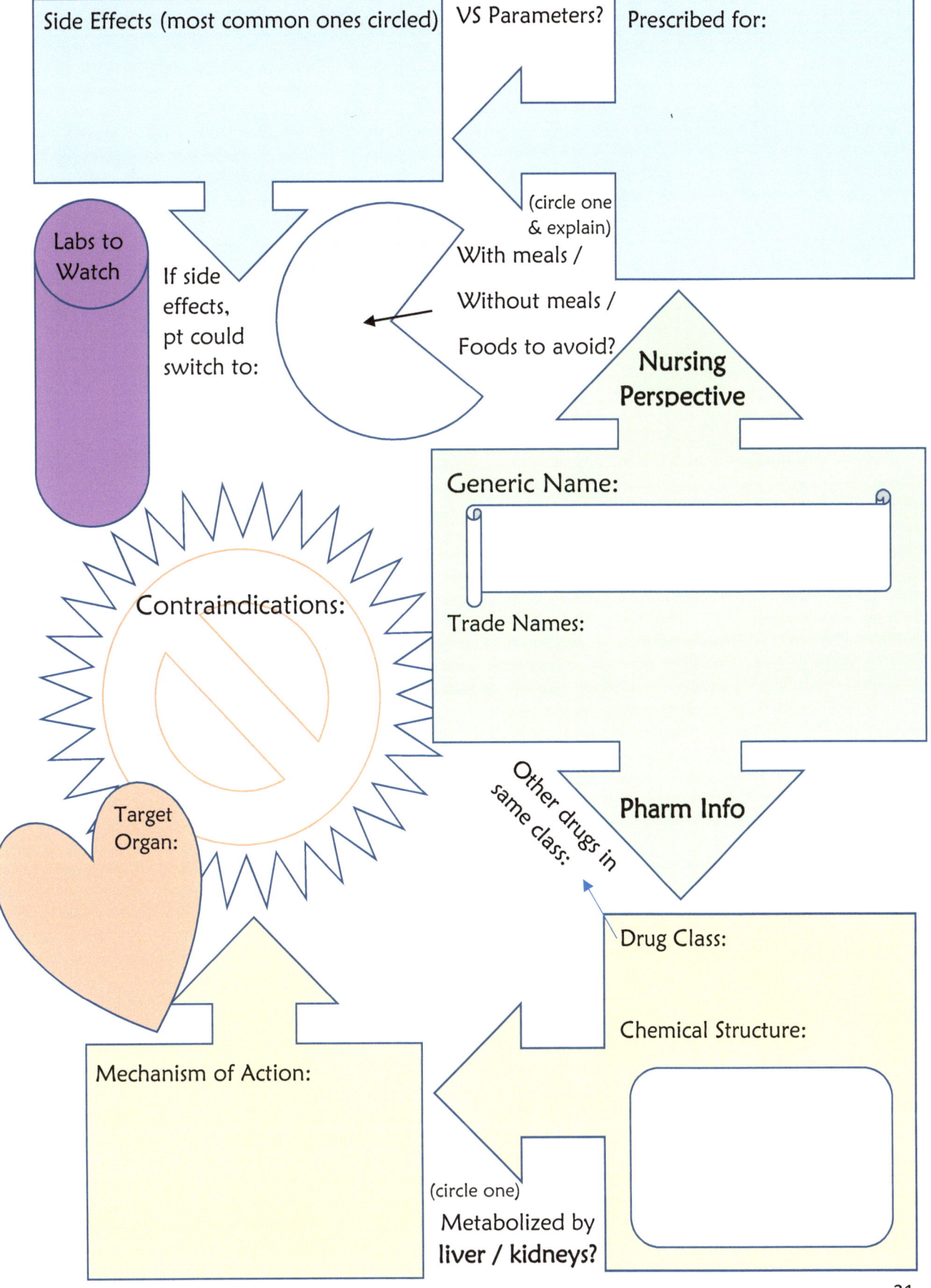

Date: Class: This content will appear on Exam #:

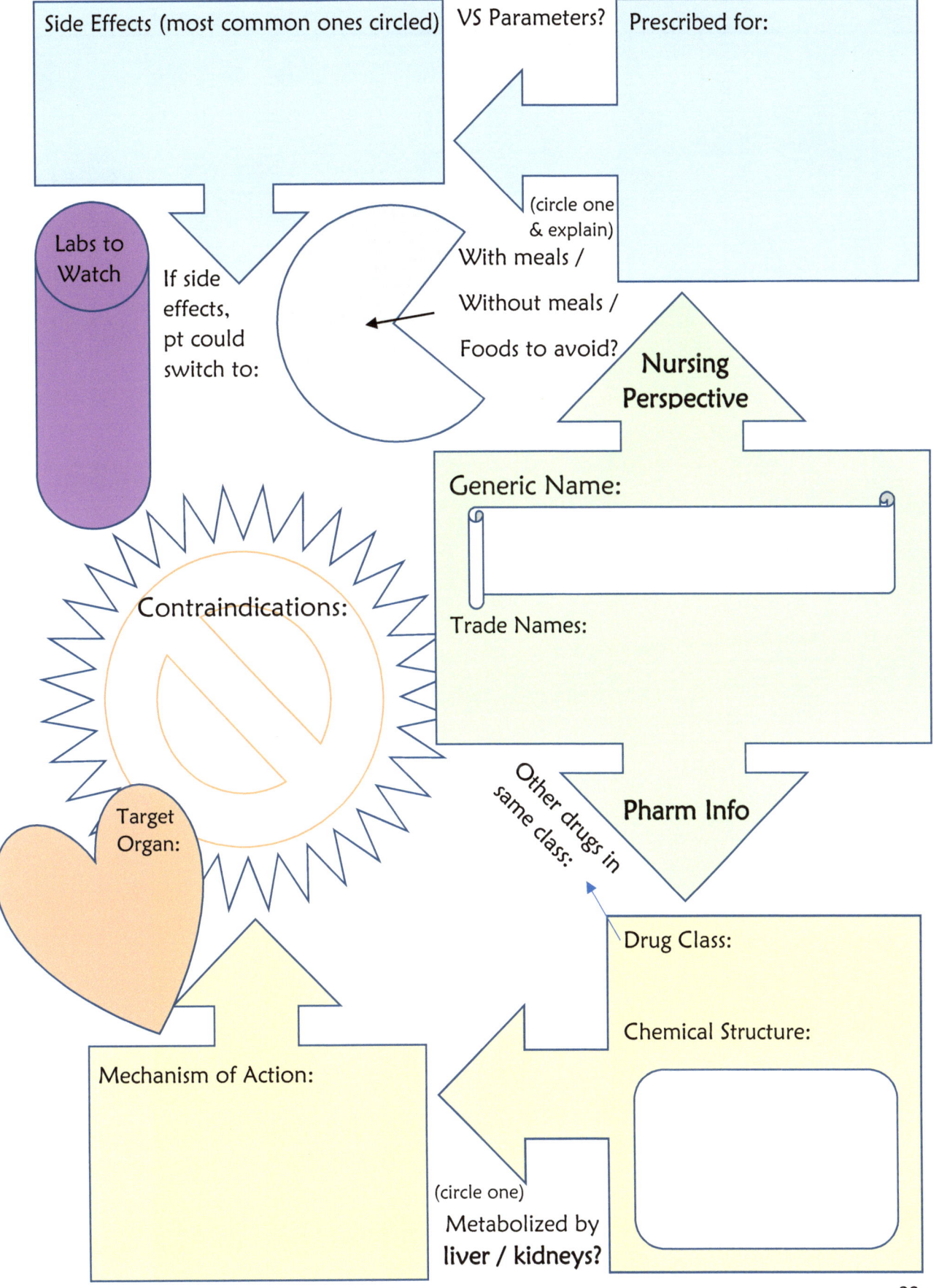

Date:　　　　　Class:　　　　　　　　This content will appear on Exam #:

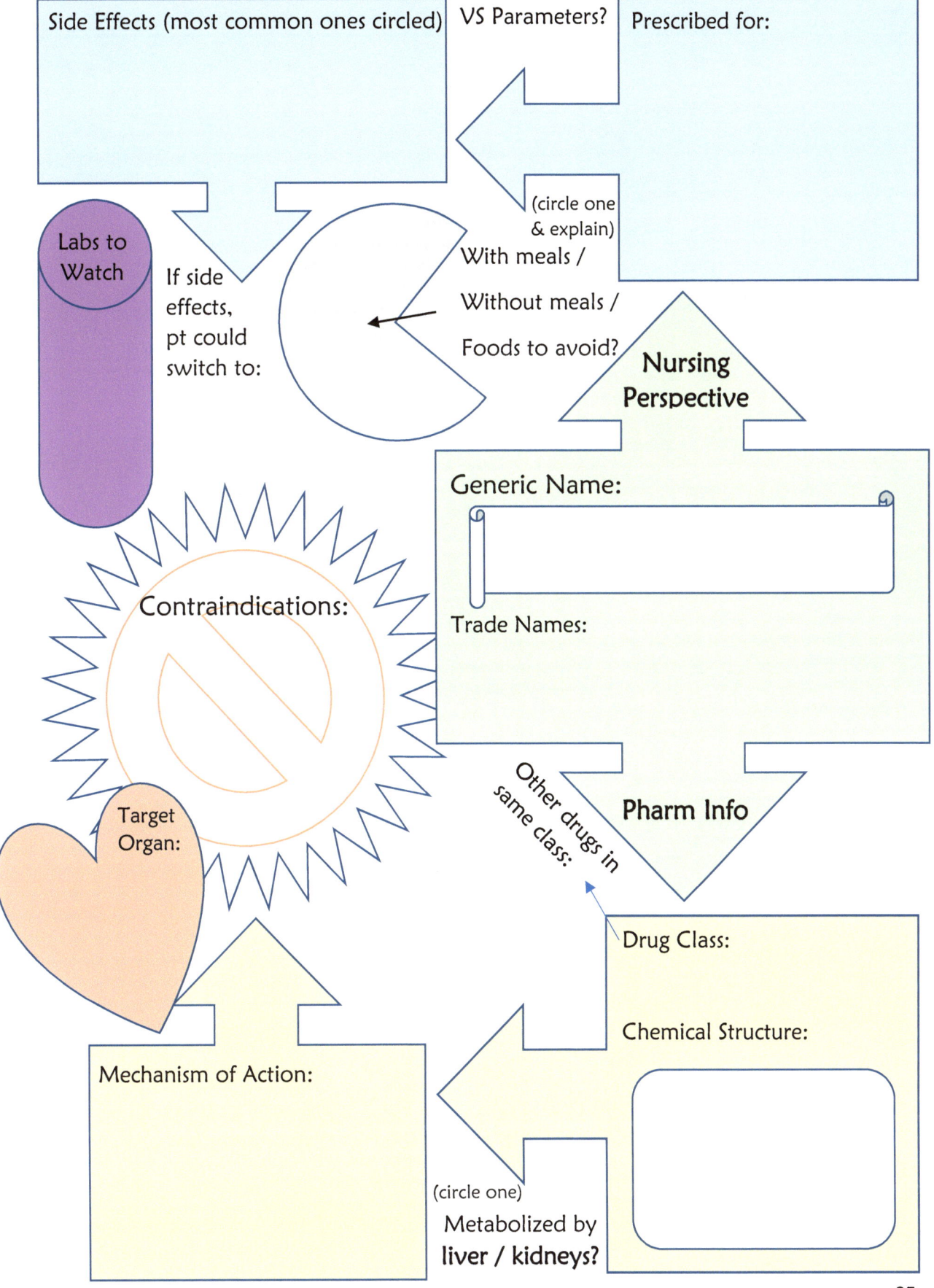

Date: Class: This content will appear on Exam #:

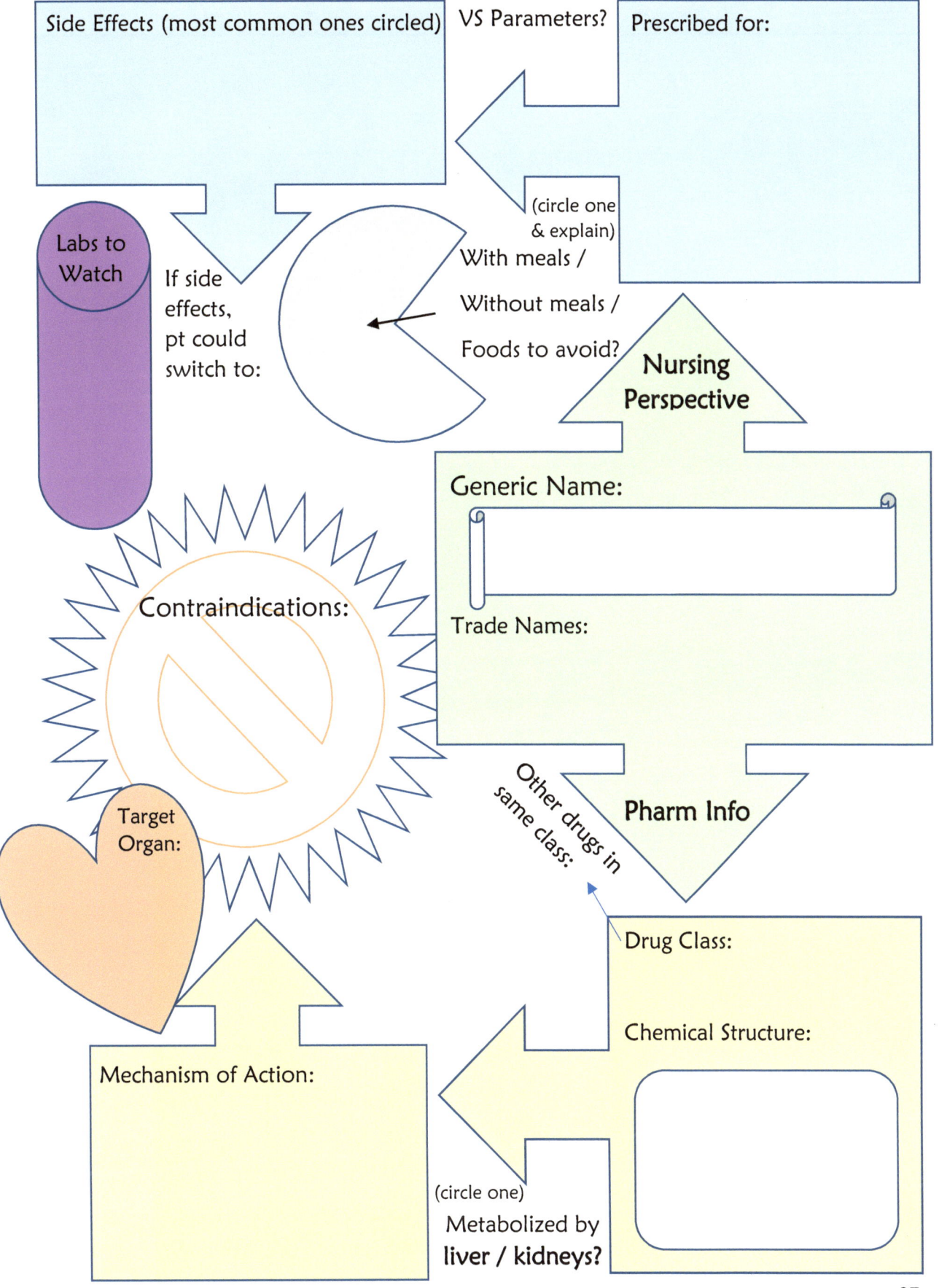

Date:　　　　　　　Class:　　　　　　　　　This content will appear on Exam #:

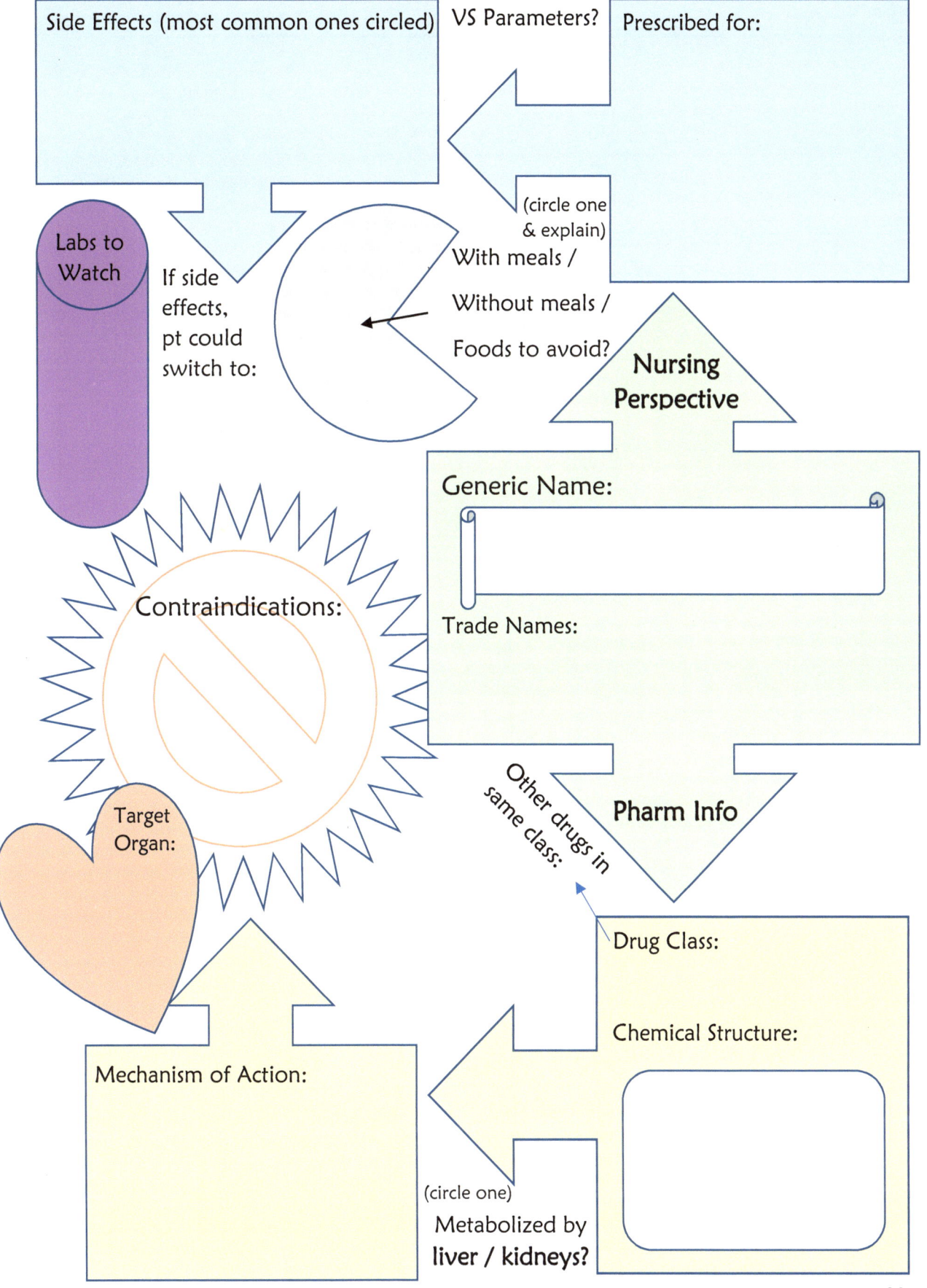

Date: Class: This content will appear on Exam #:

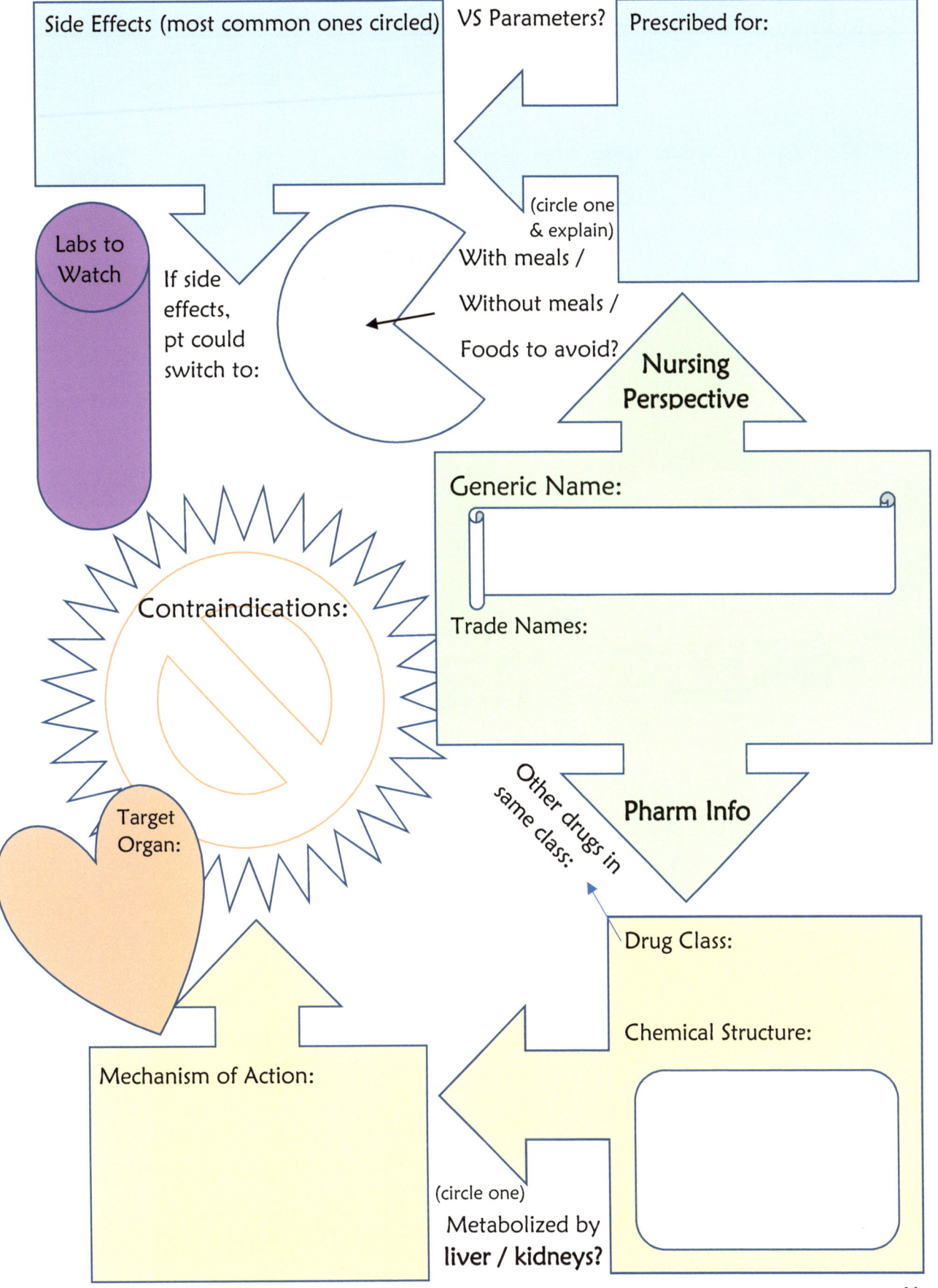

Date: Class: This content will appear on Exam #:

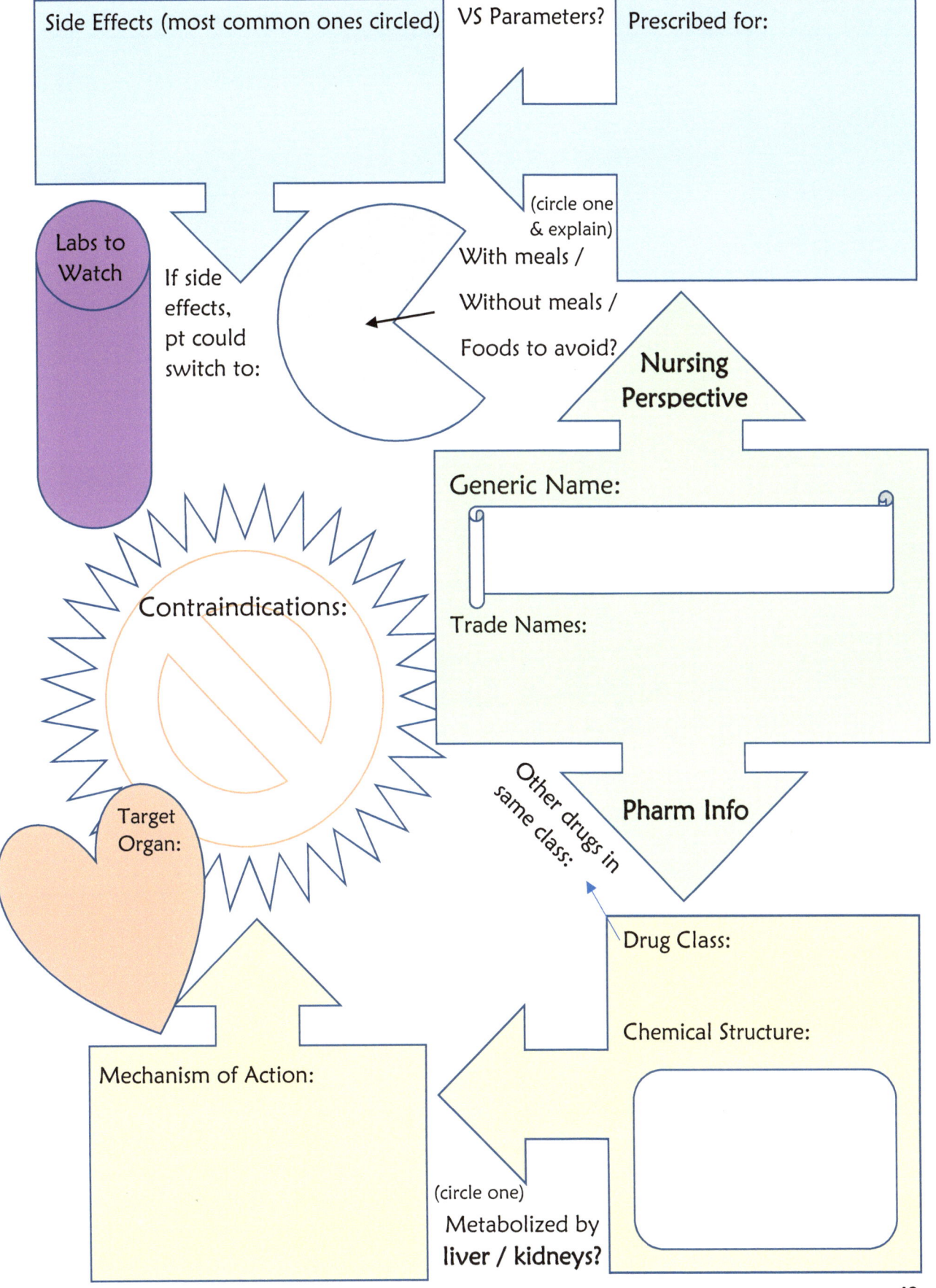

Date: Class: This content will appear on Exam #:

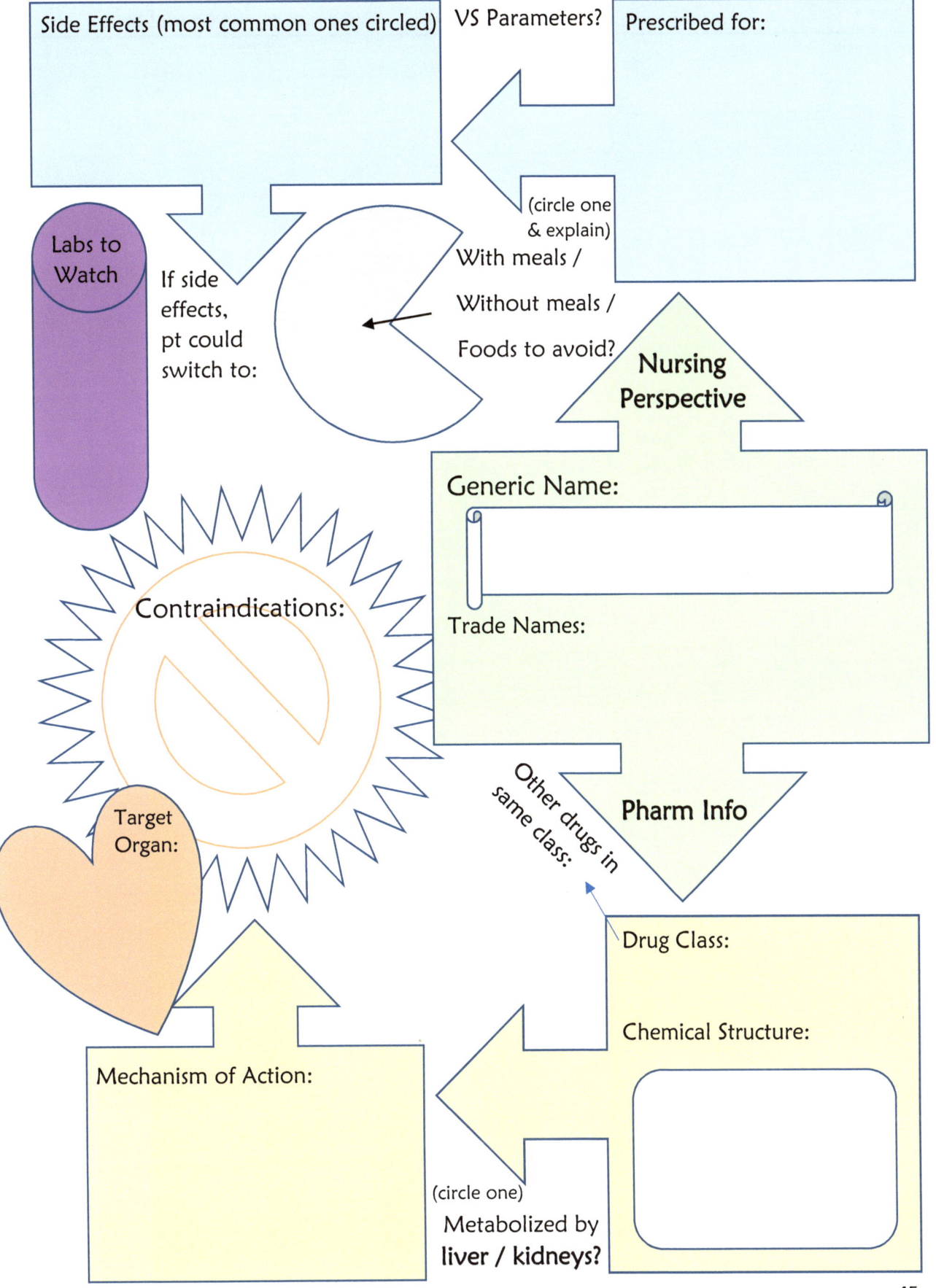

Date: Class: This content will appear on Exam #:

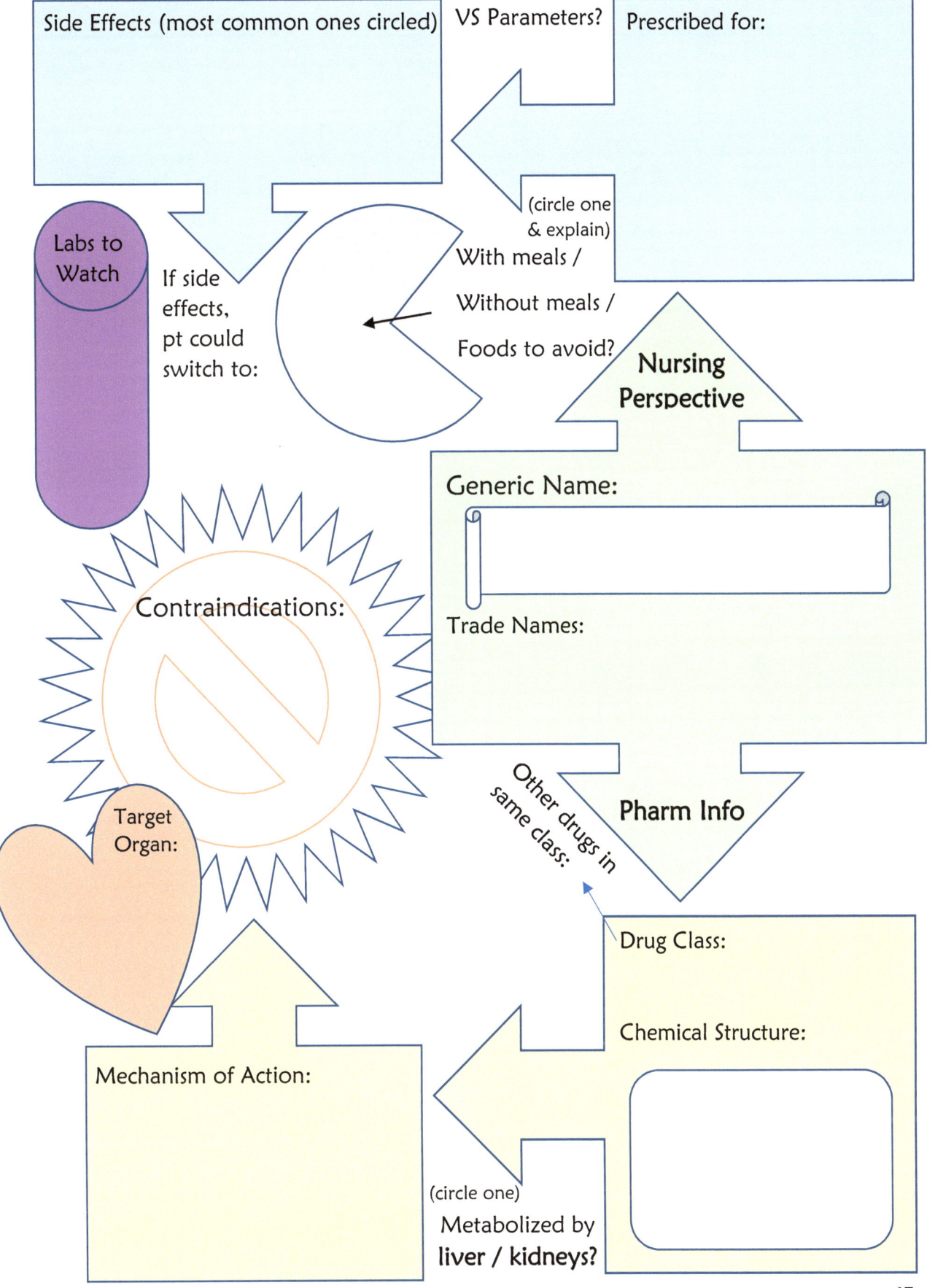

Date: Class: This content will appear on Exam #:

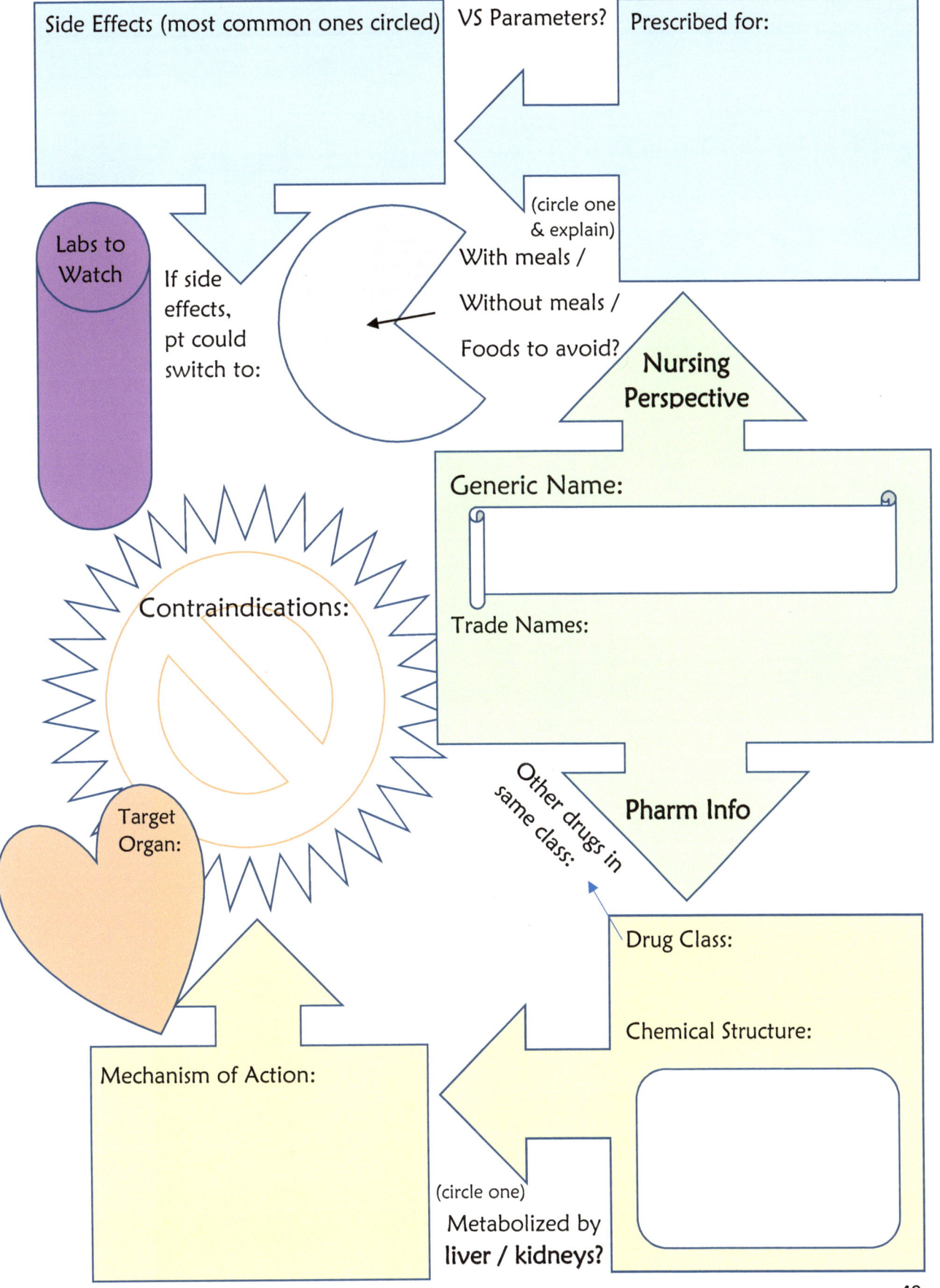

Date: Class: This content will appear on Exam #:

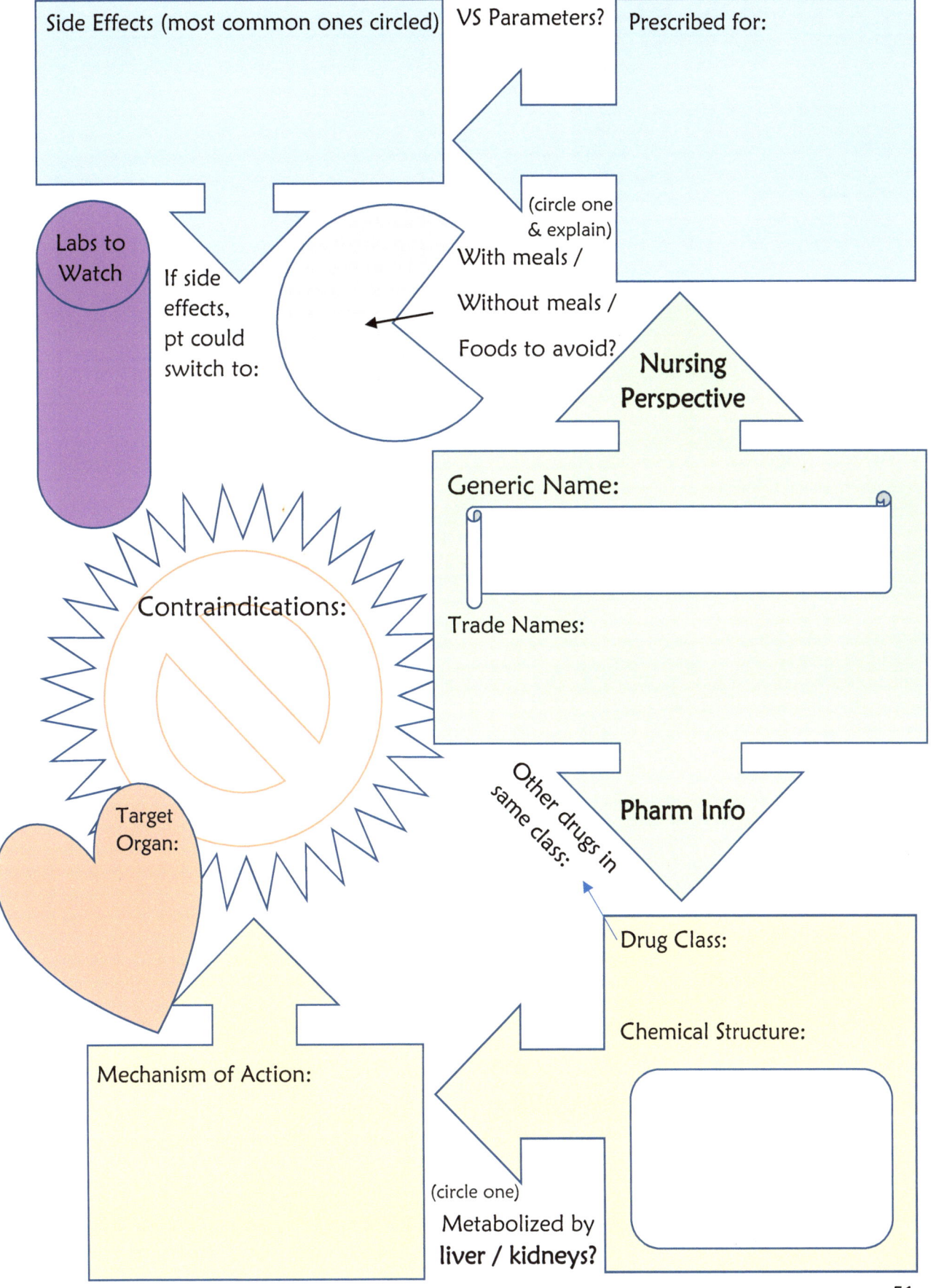

Date: Class: This content will appear on Exam #:

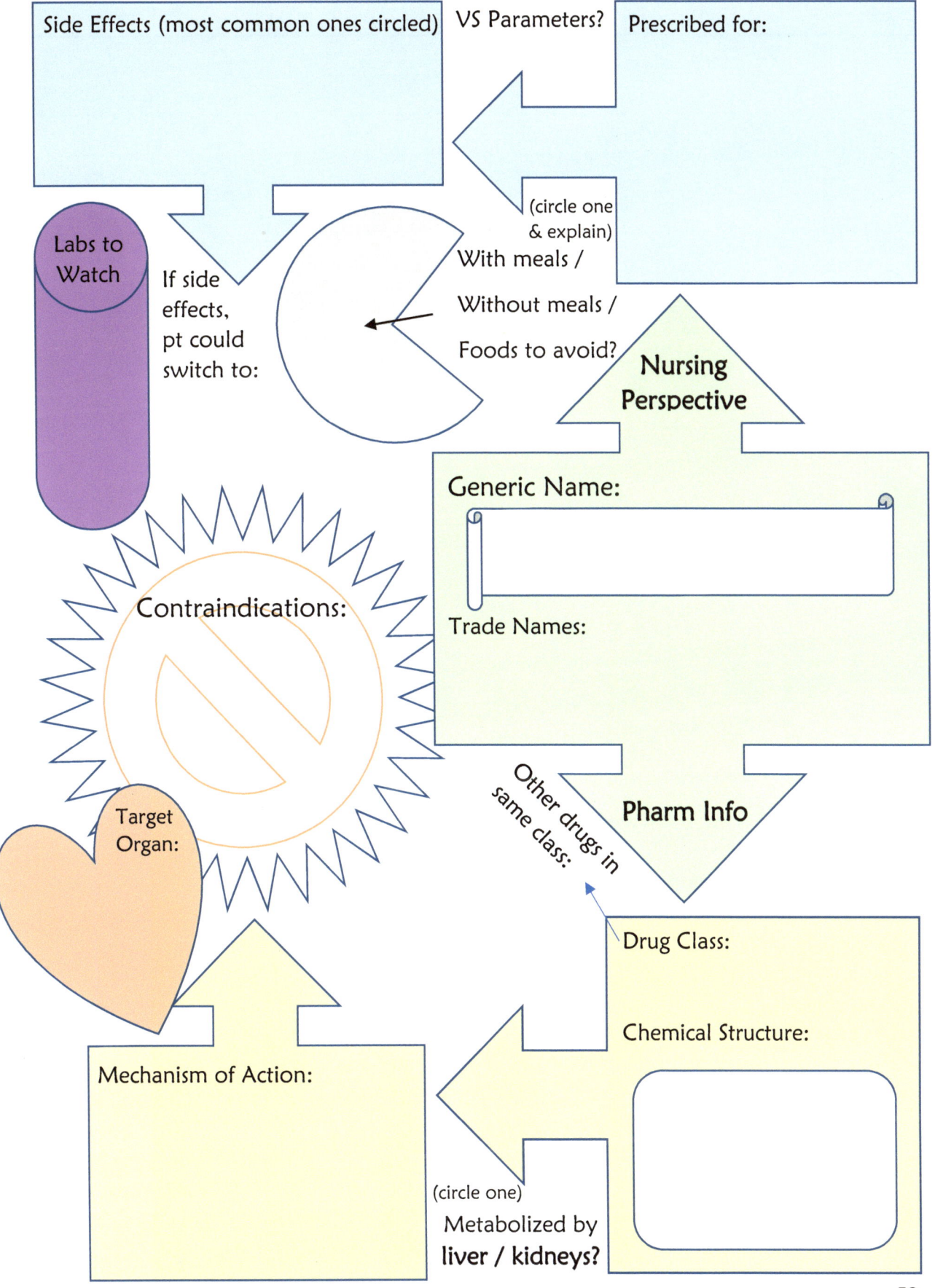

Date: Class: This content will appear on Exam #:

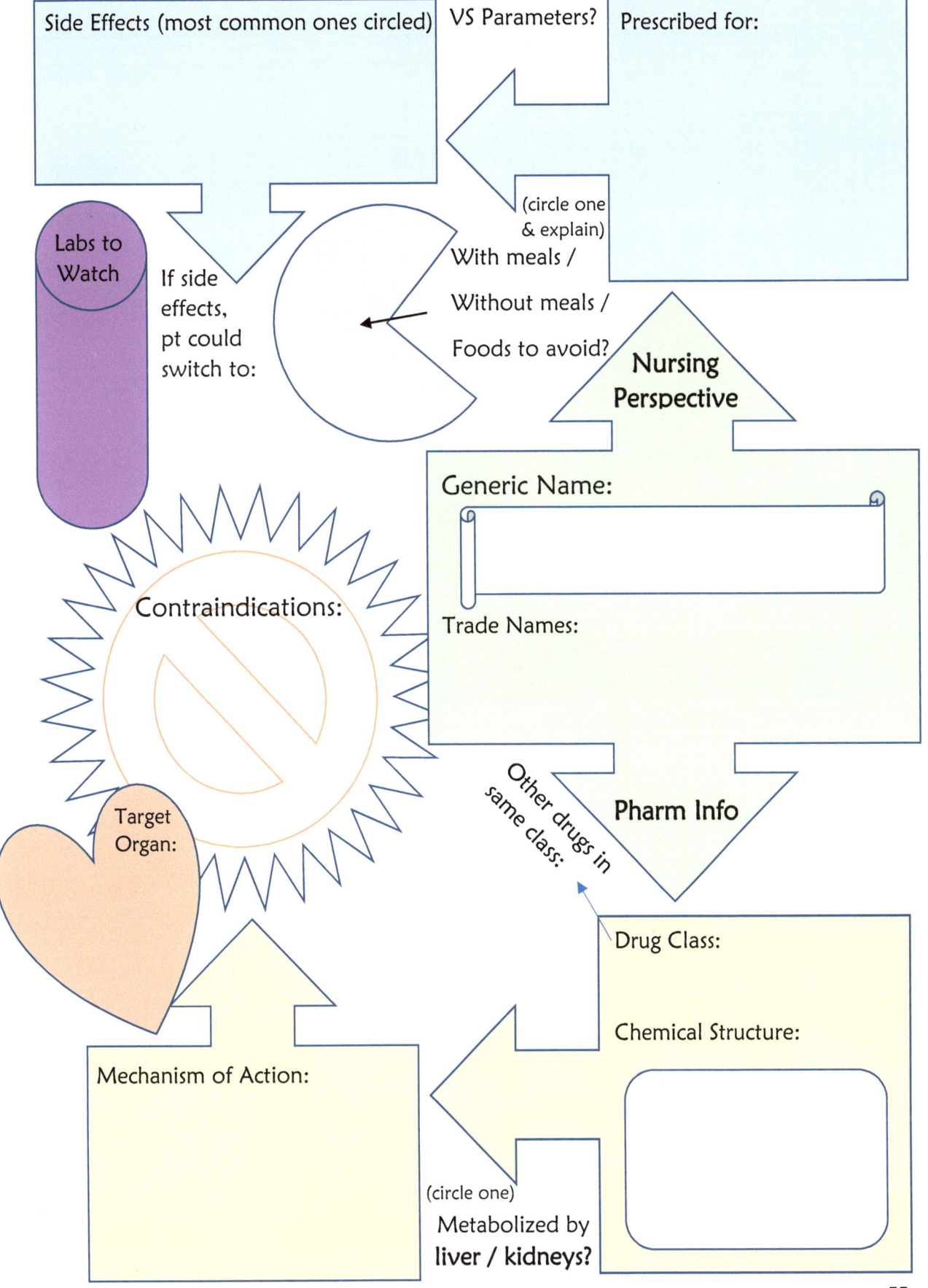

Date: Class: This content will appear on Exam #:

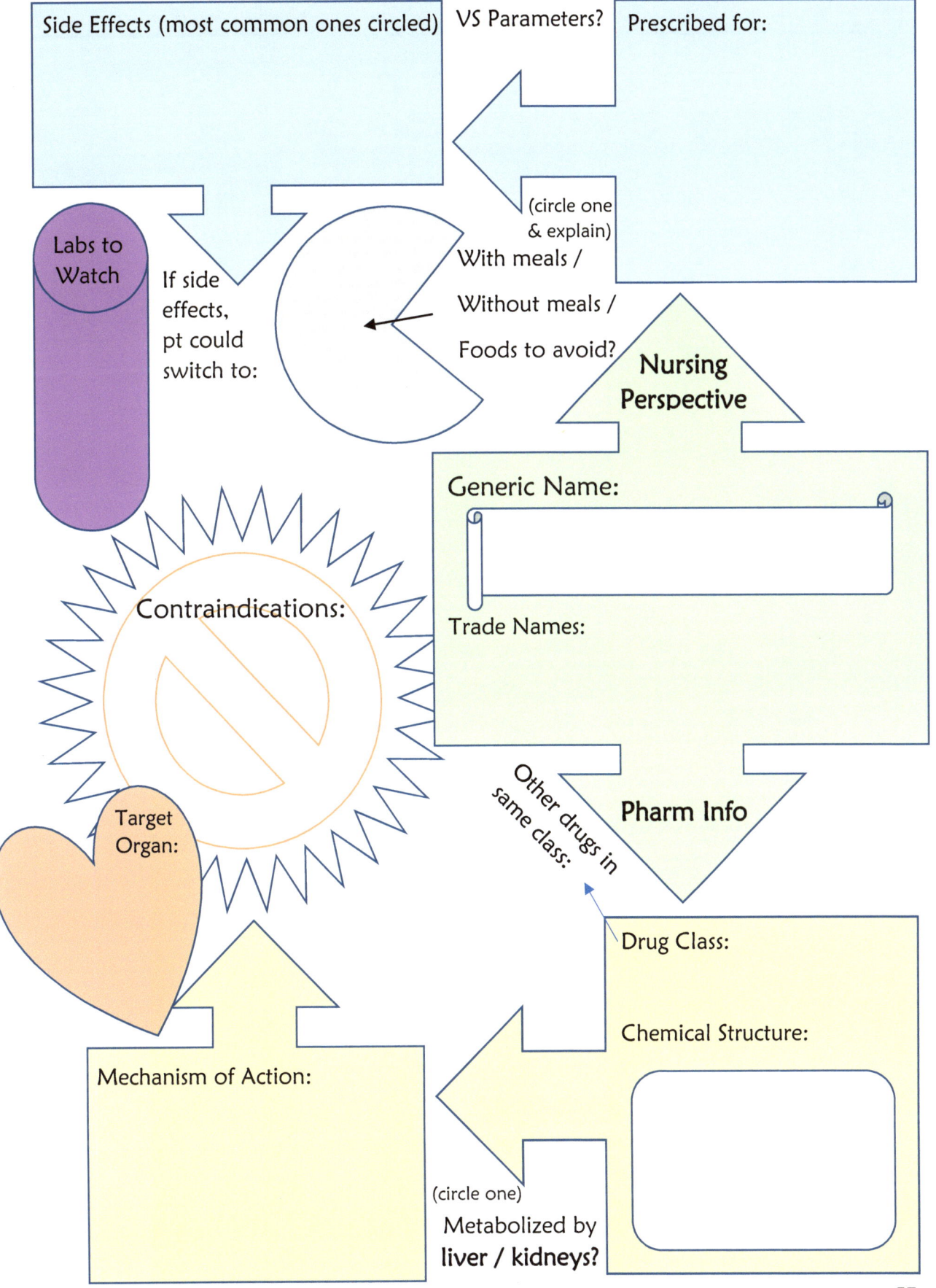

Date:	Class:	This content will appear on Exam #:

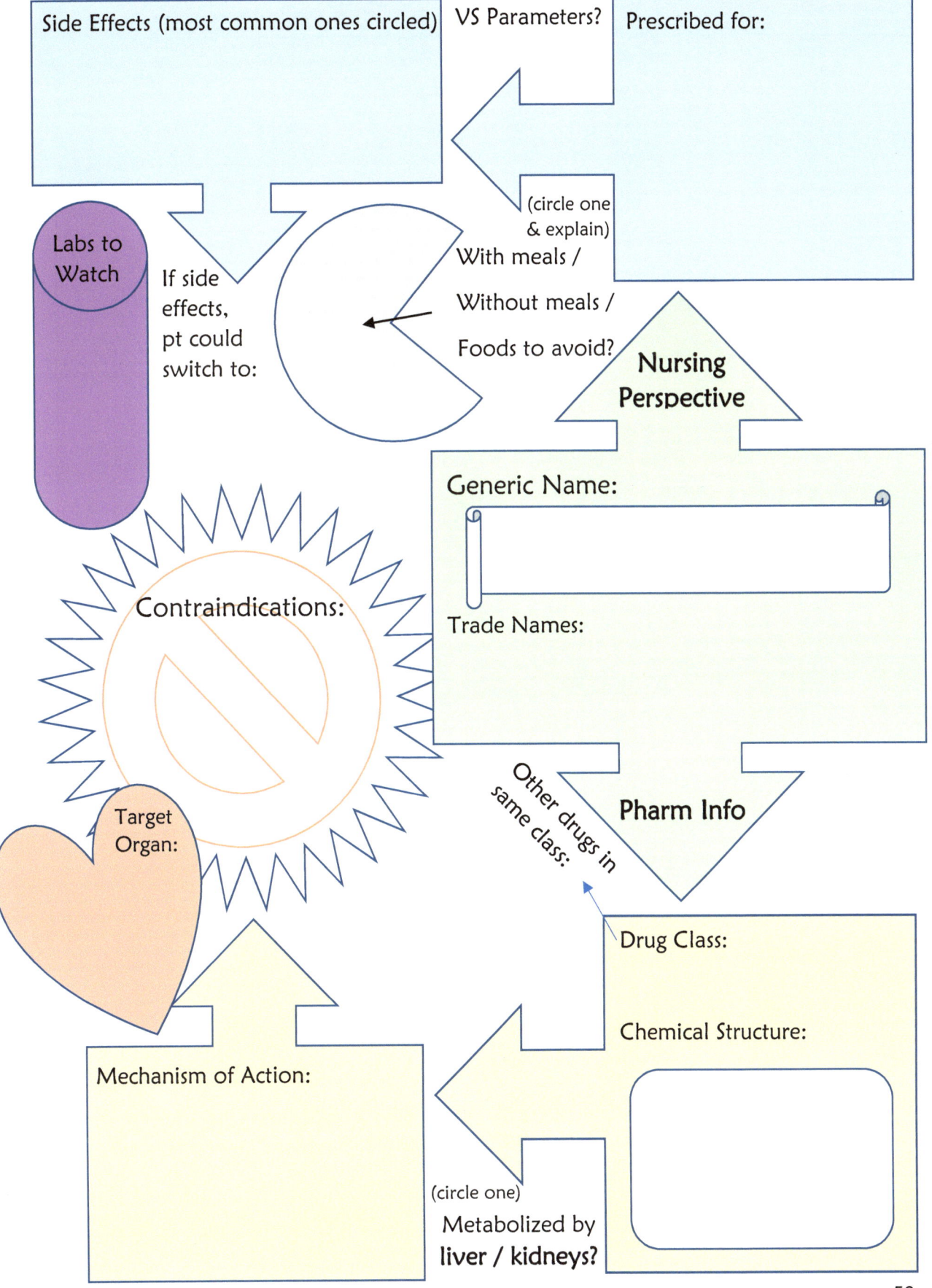

Date: Class: This content will appear on Exam #:

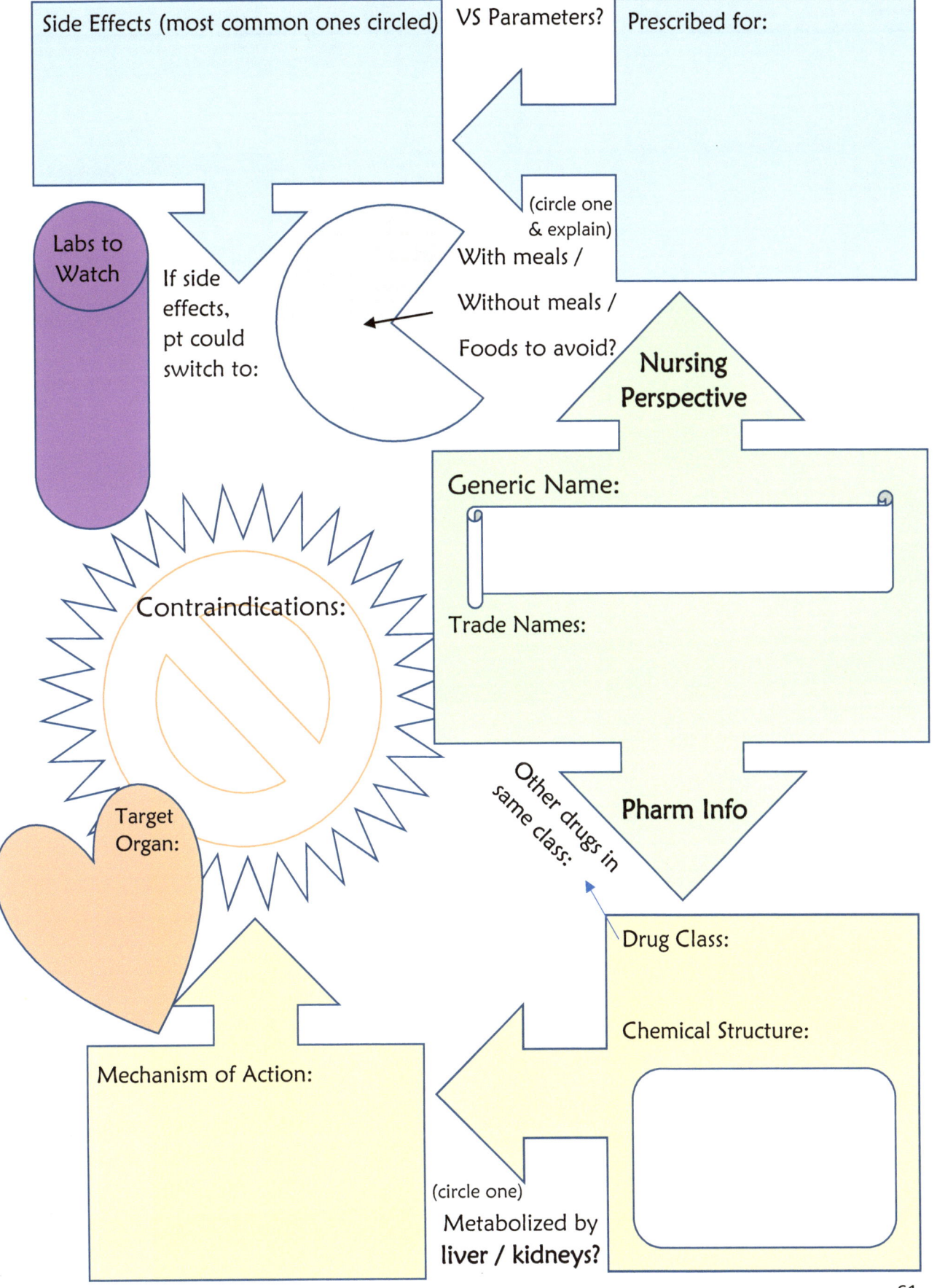

Date: Class: This content will appear on Exam #:

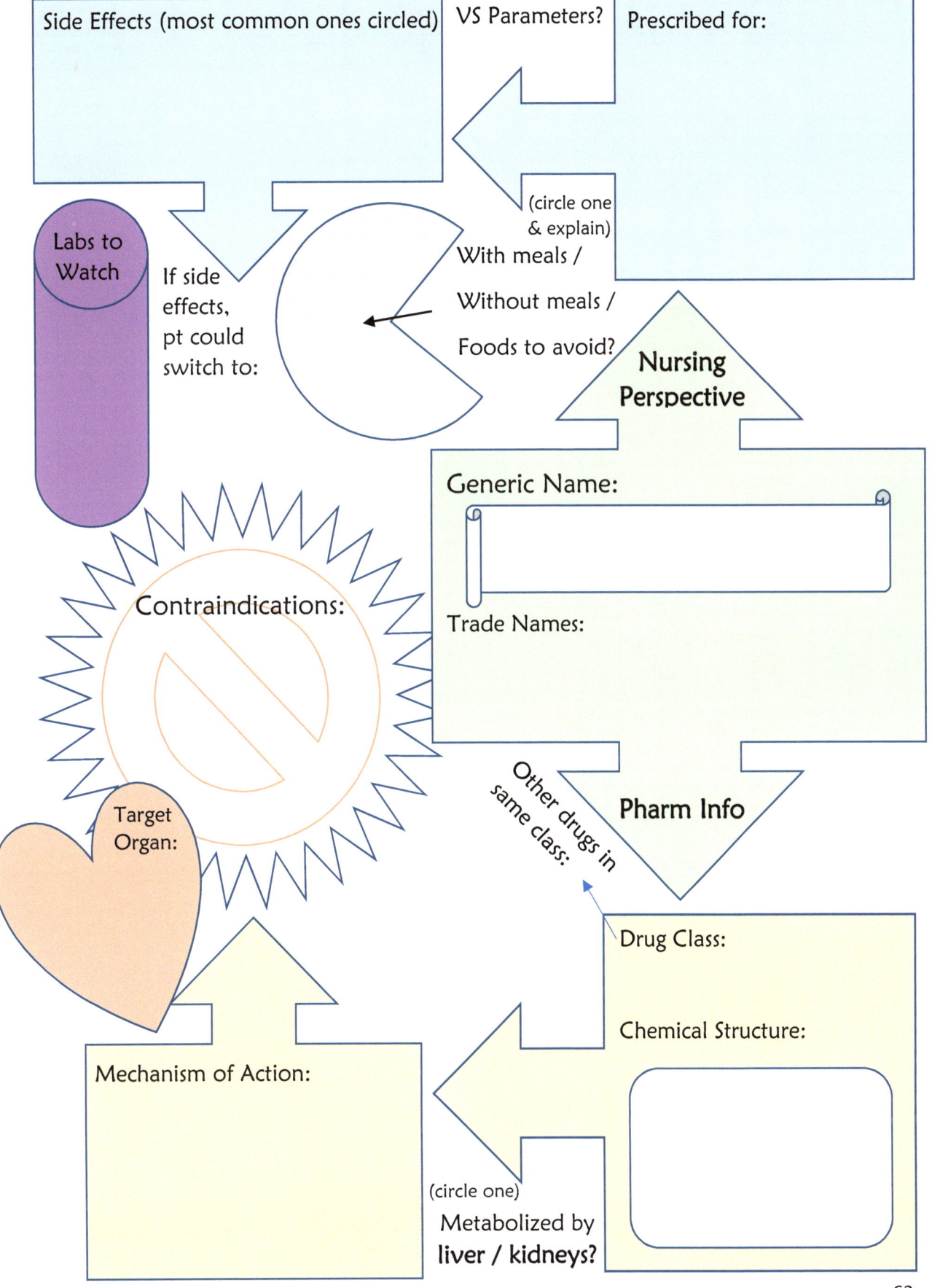

Date: Class: This content will appear on Exam #:

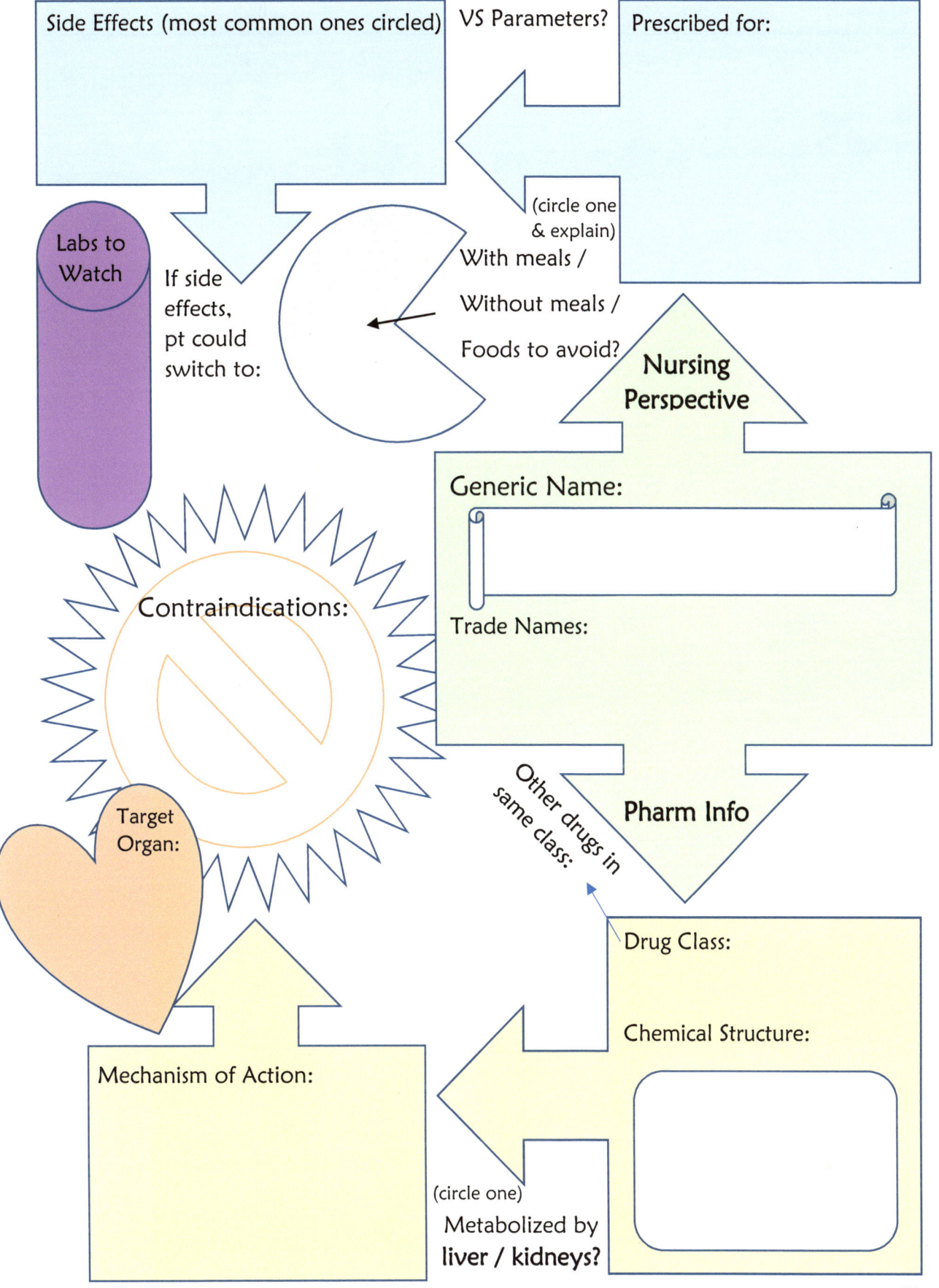

Date: Class: This content will appear on Exam #:

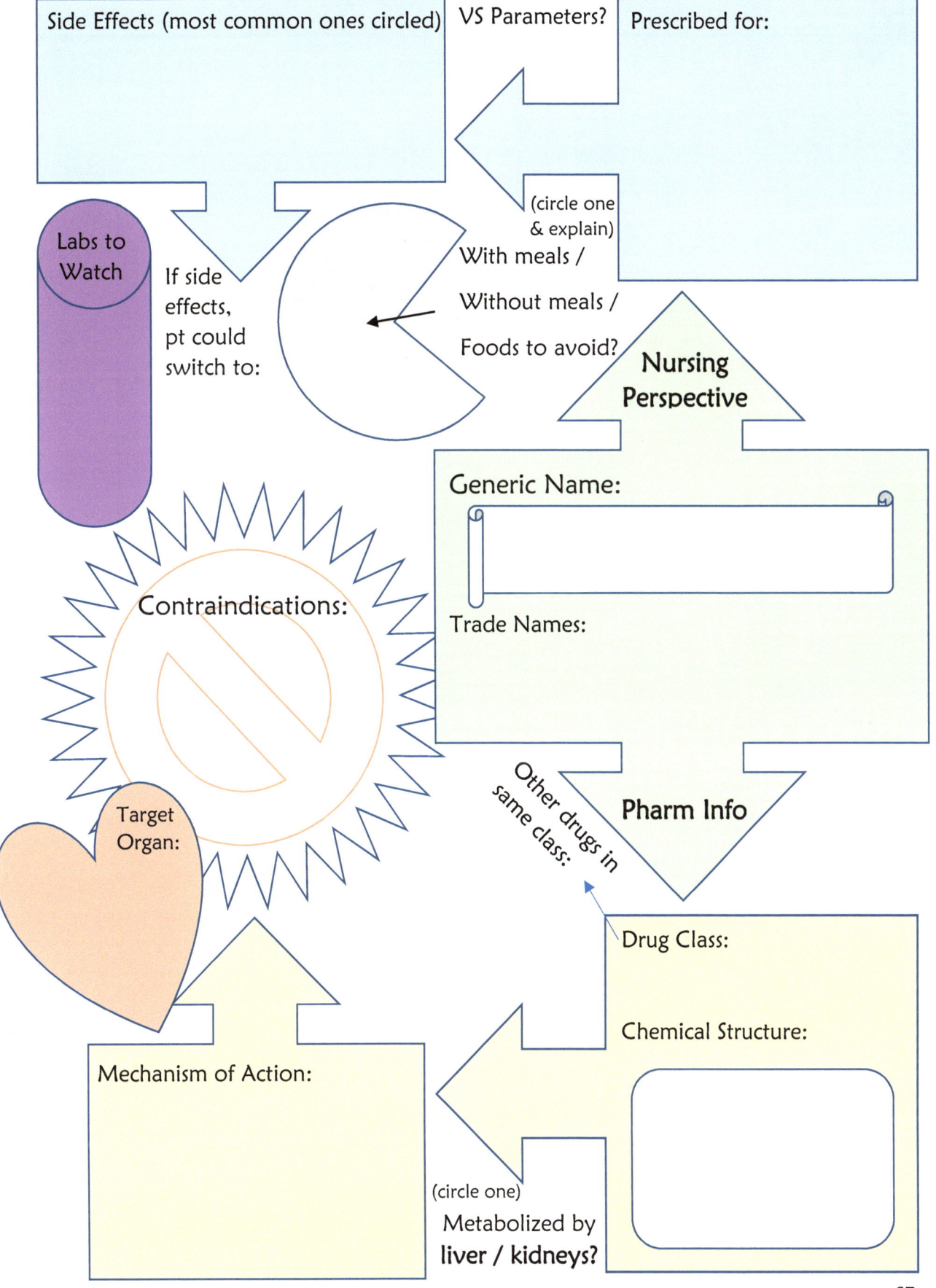

Date: Class: This content will appear on Exam #:

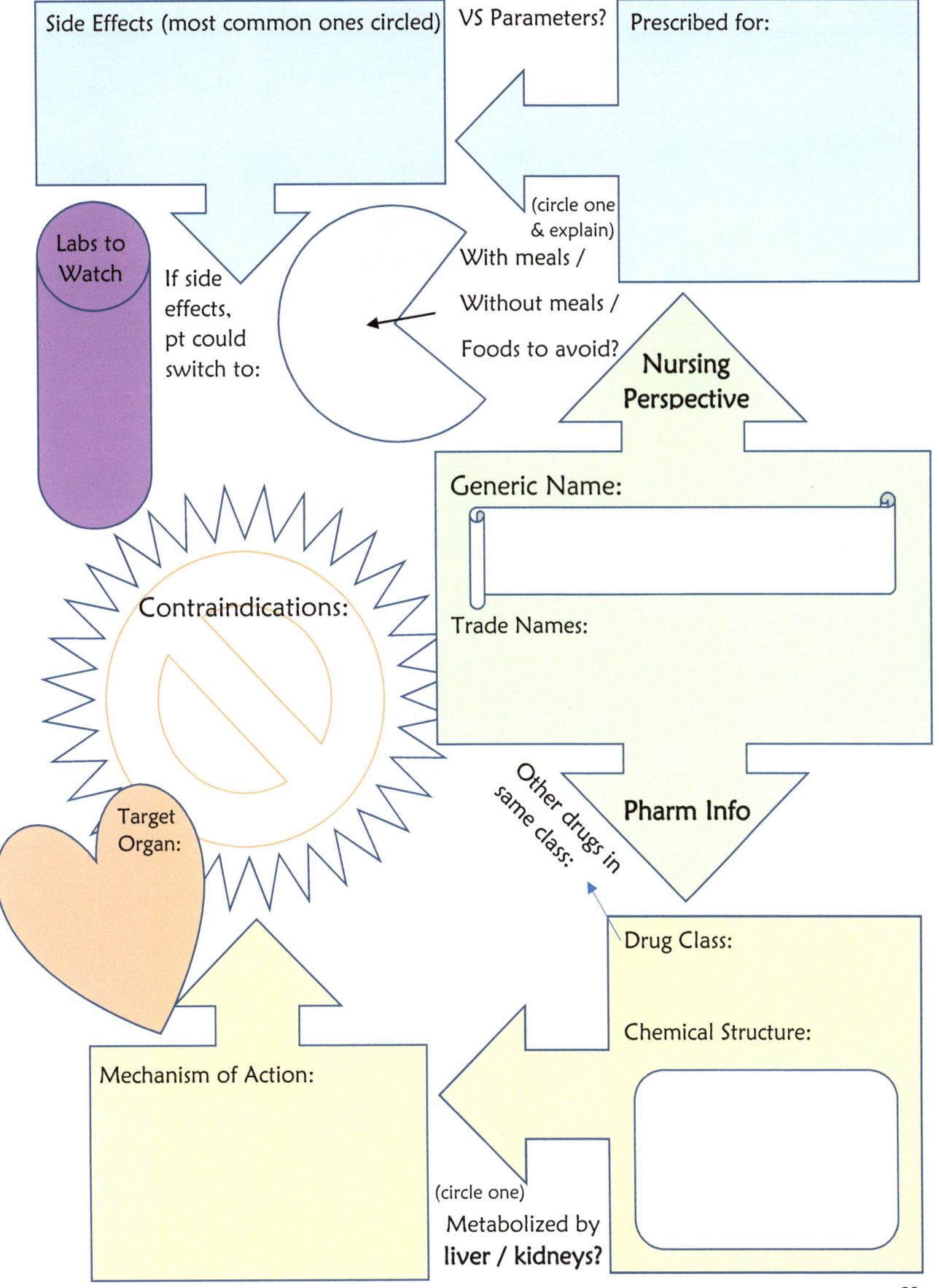

Date: Class: This content will appear on Exam #:

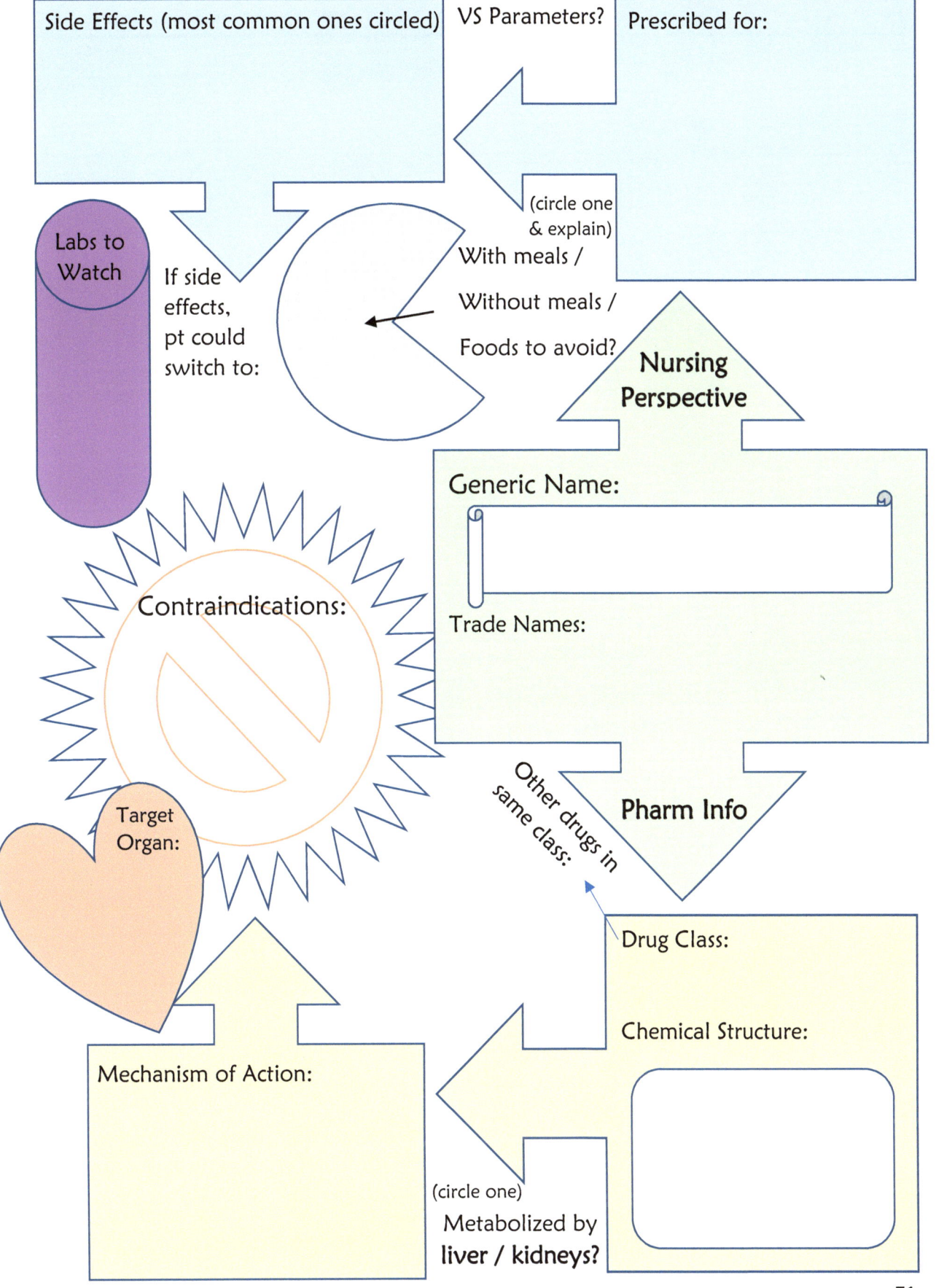

Date: Class: This content will appear on Exam #:

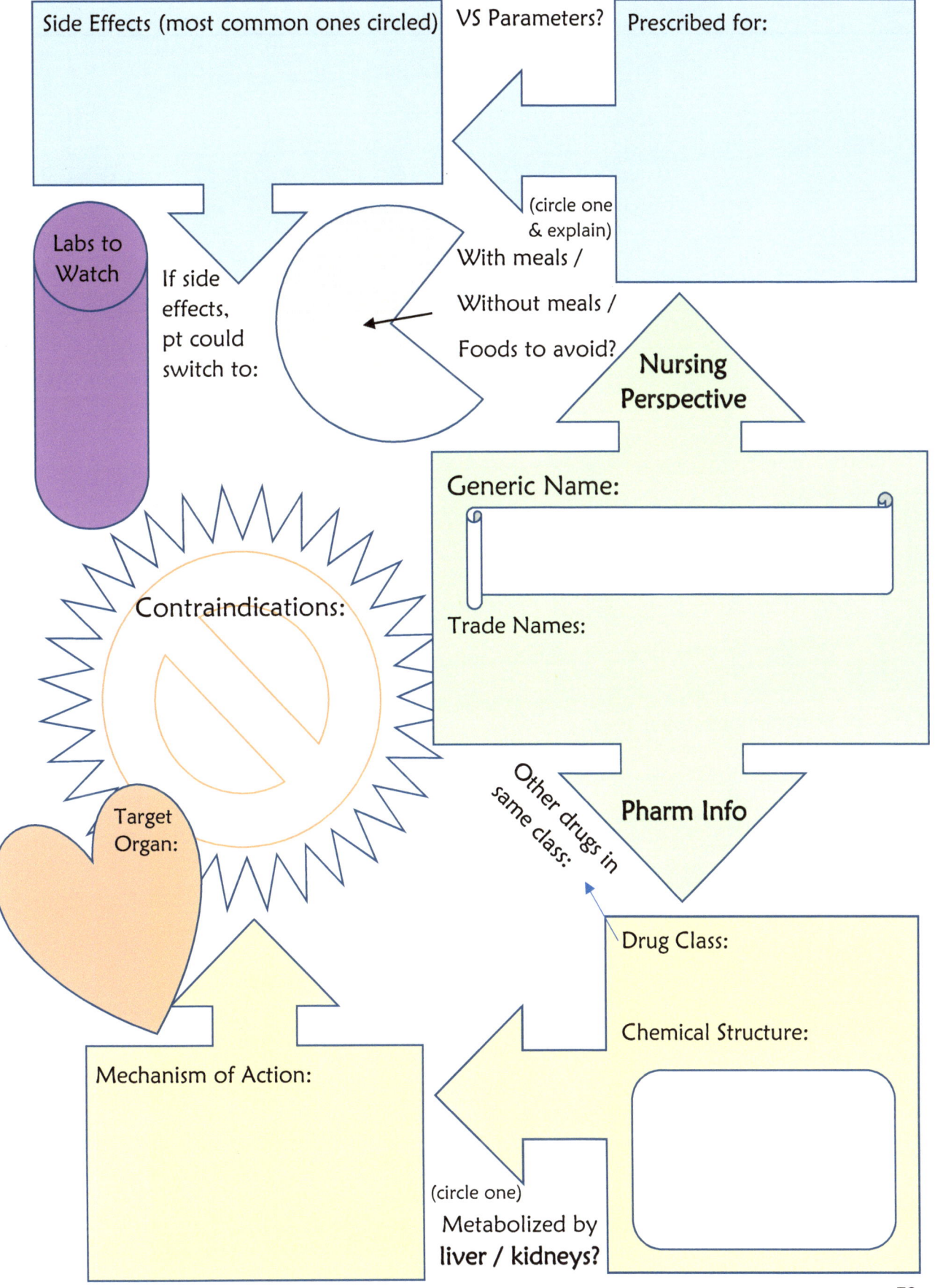

Date: Class: This content will appear on Exam #:

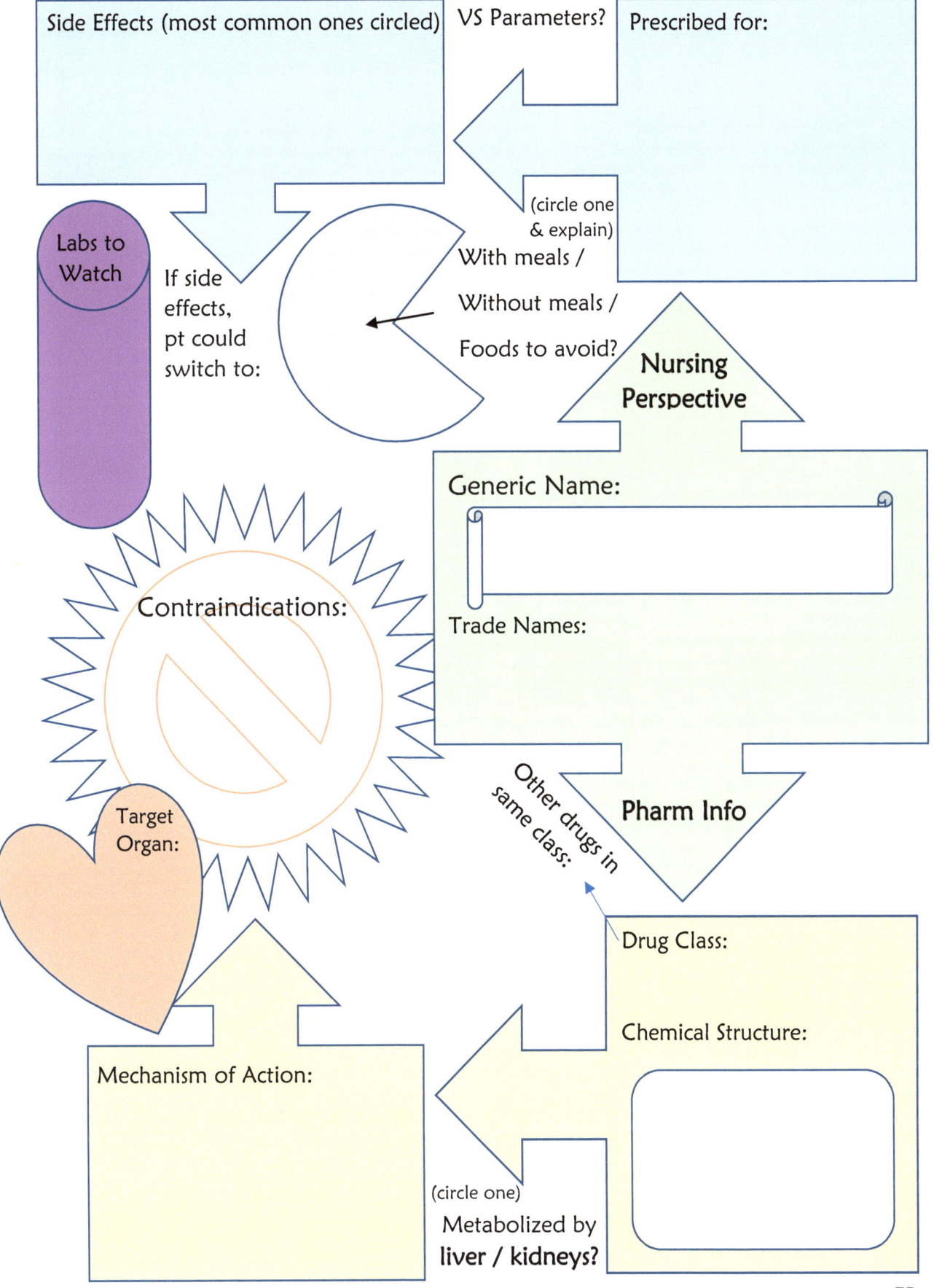

Date:	Class:	This content will appear on Exam #:

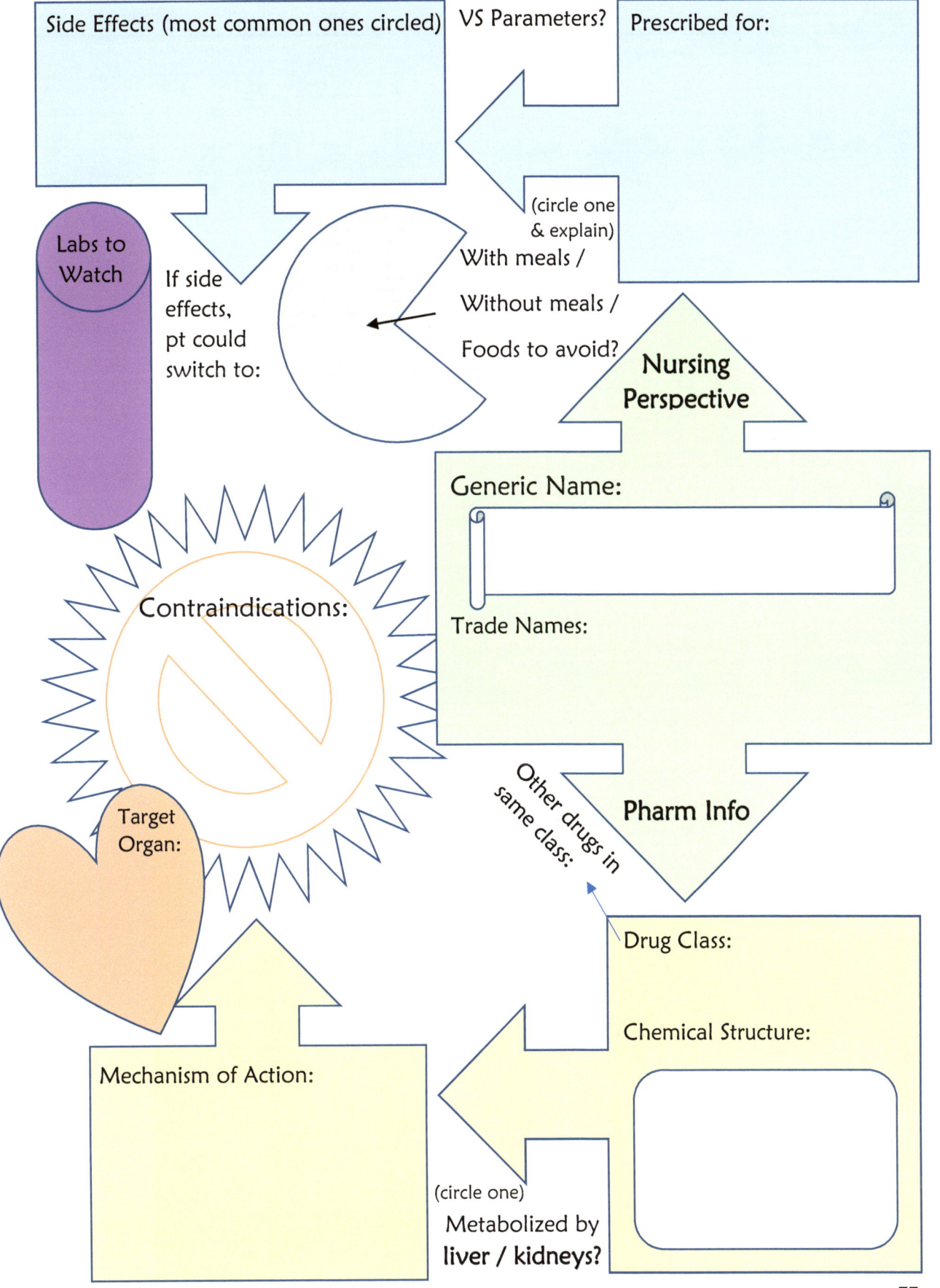

Date: Class: This content will appear on Exam #:

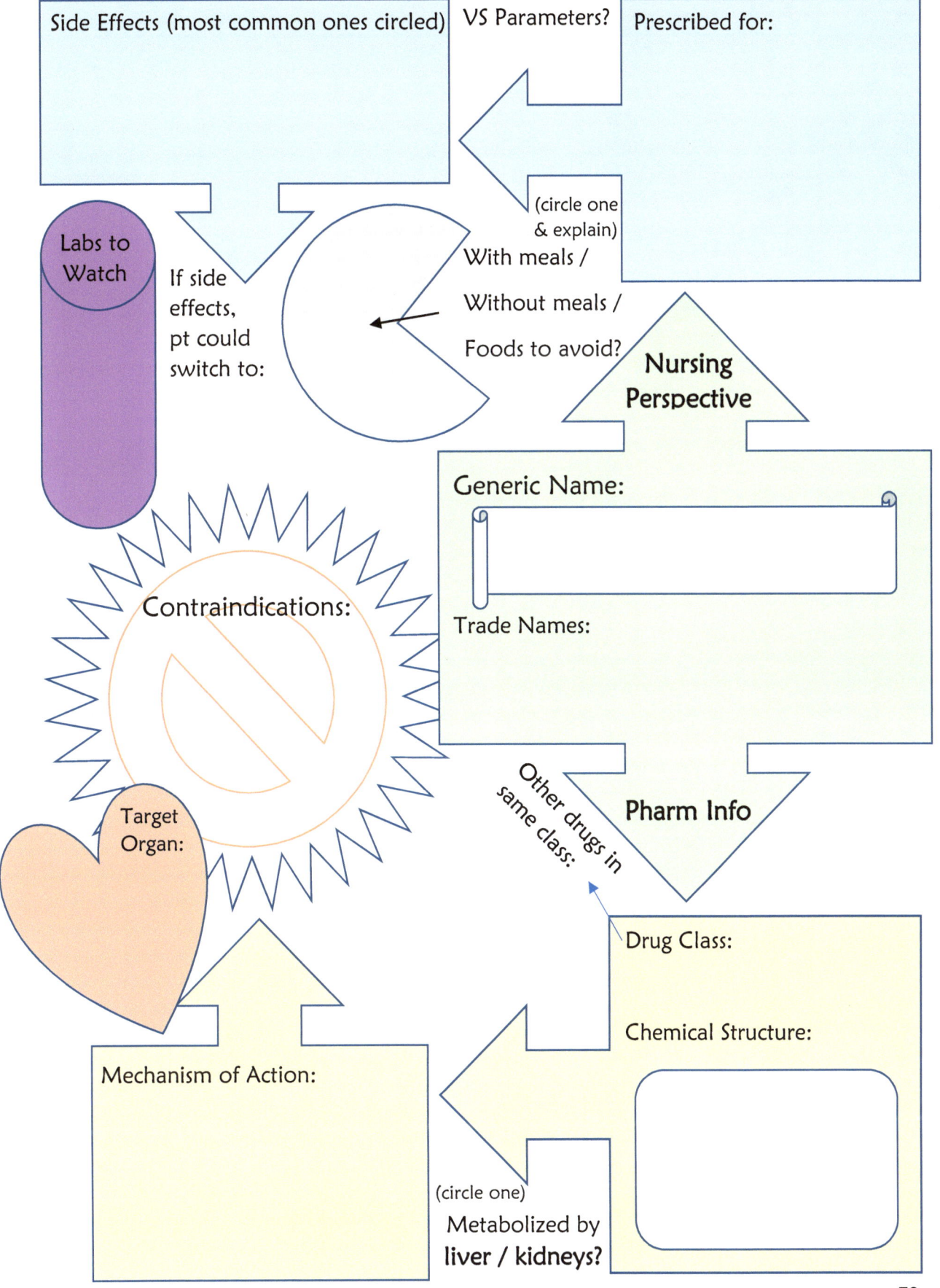

Date: Class: This content will appear on Exam #:

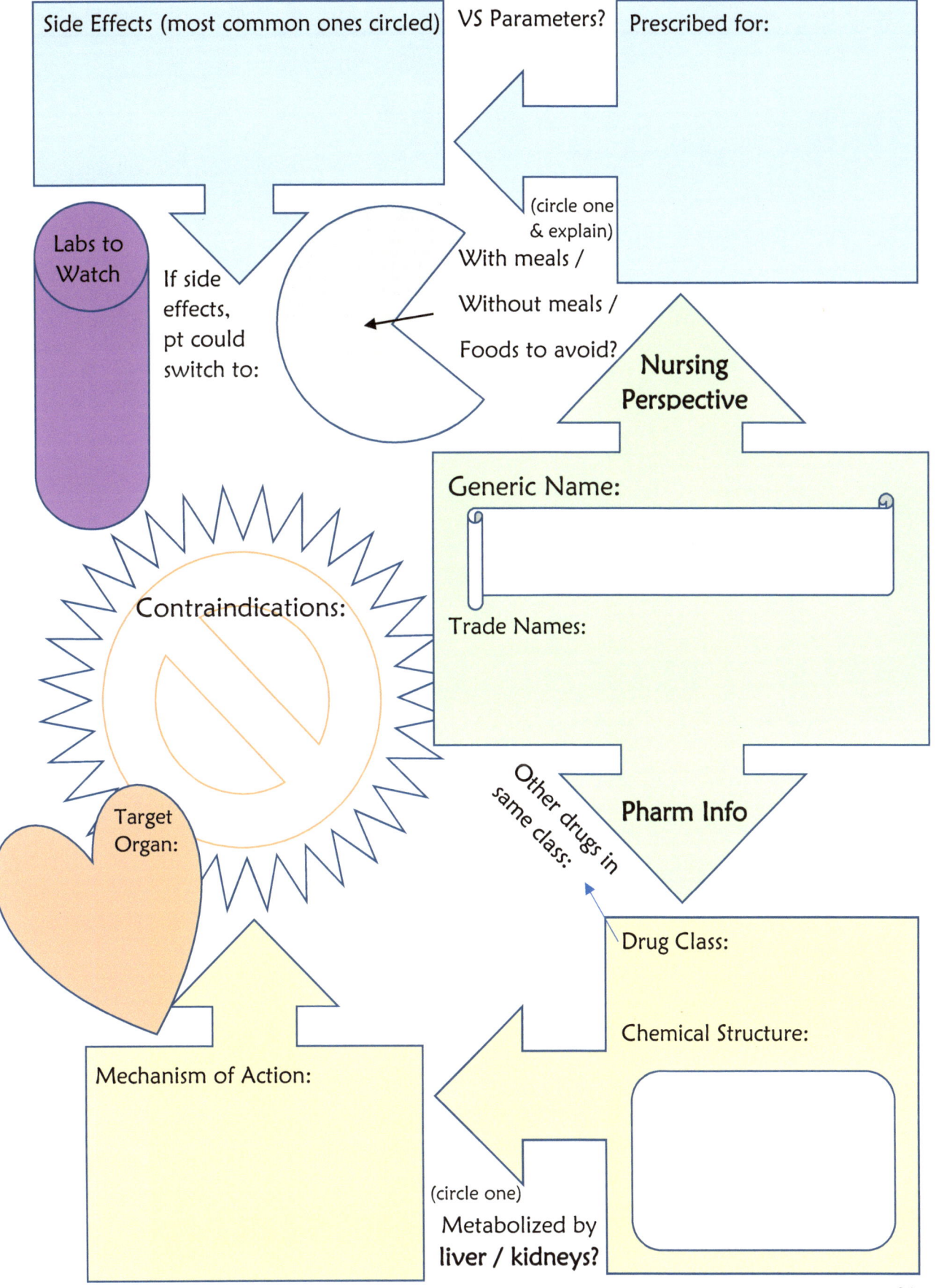

Date: Class: This content will appear on Exam #:

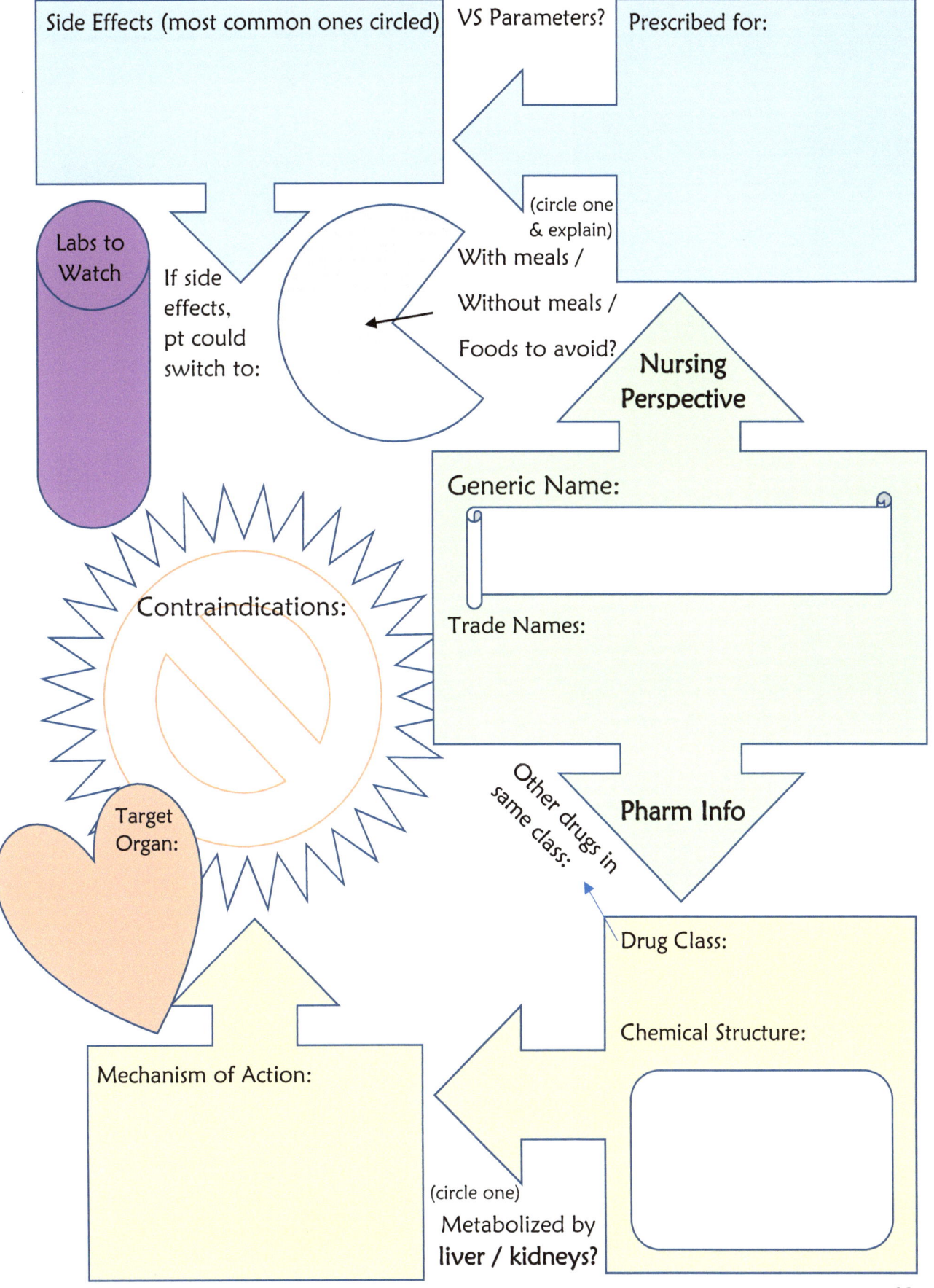

Date: Class: This content will appear on Exam #:

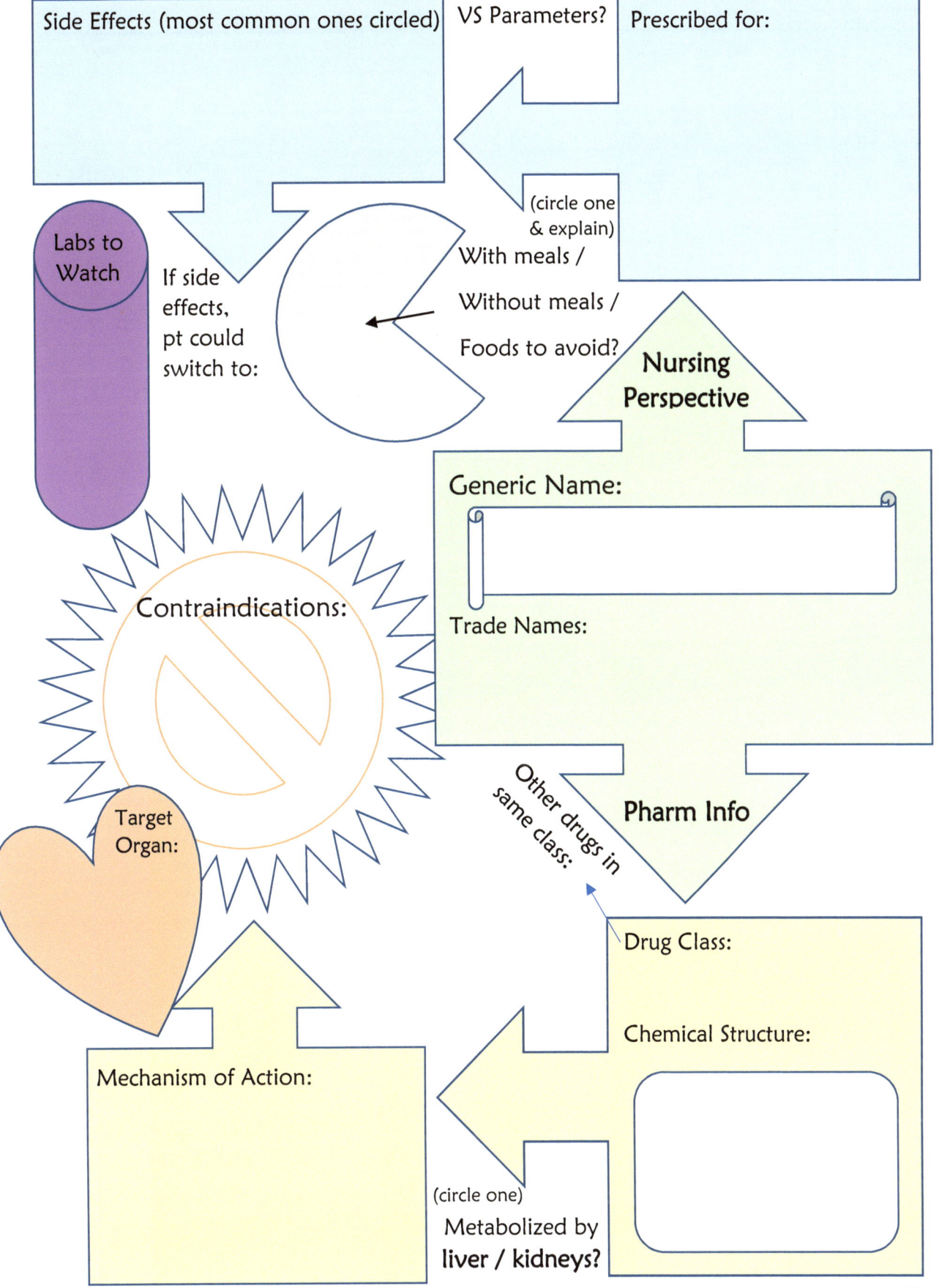

Date: Class: This content will appear on Exam #:

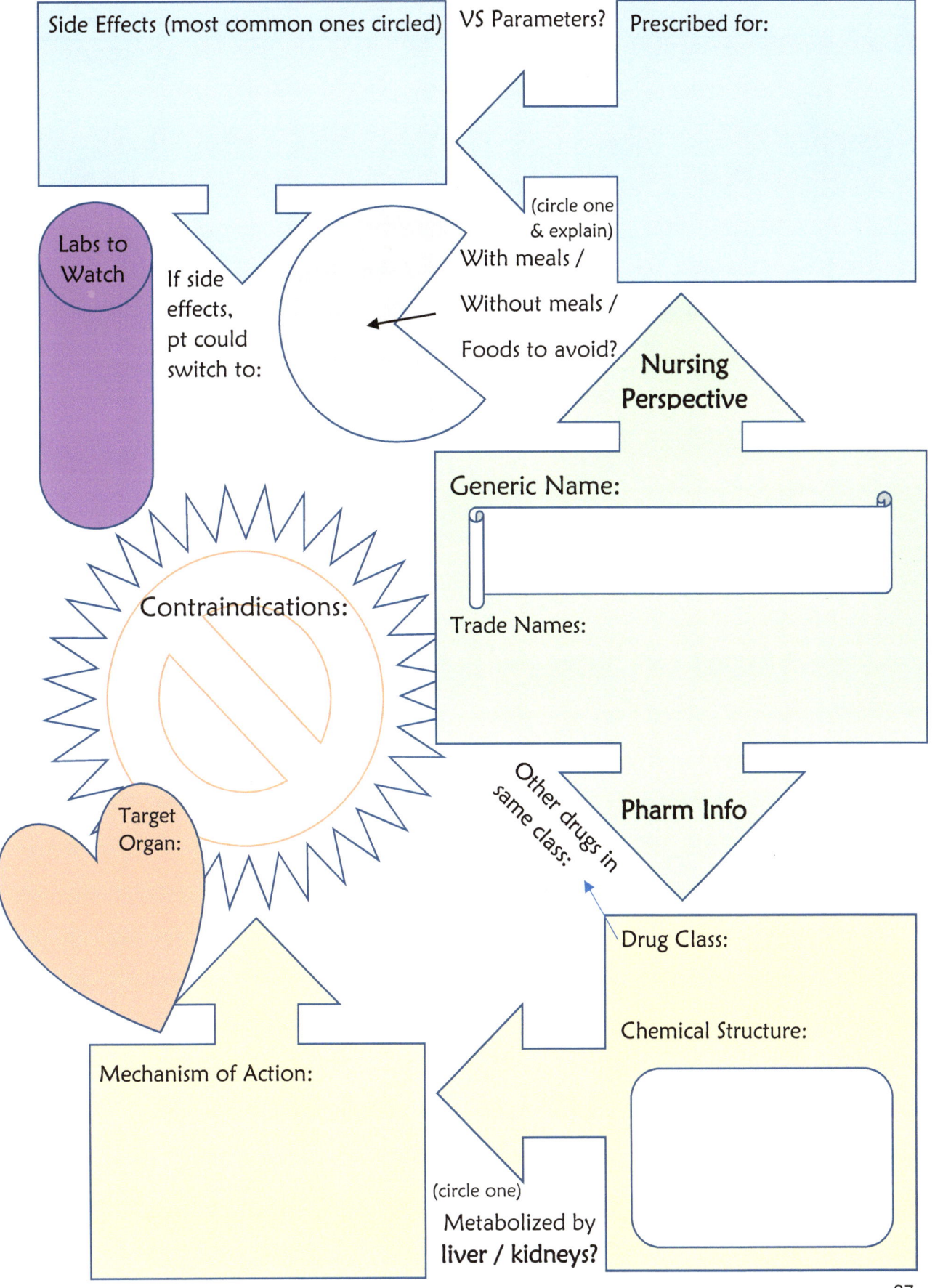

Date:　　　　　　Class:　　　　　　　　　　This content will appear on Exam #:

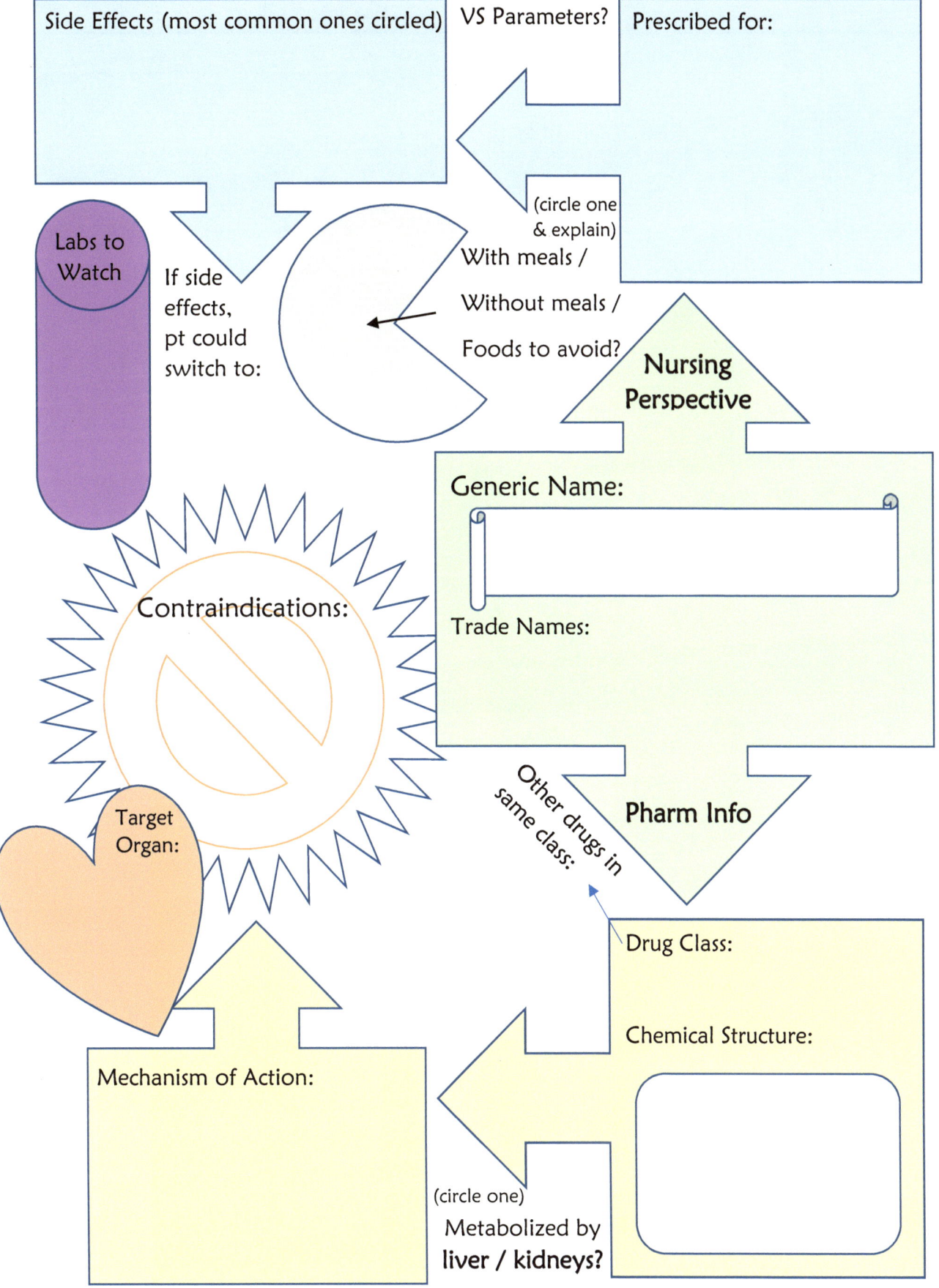

Date: Class: This content will appear on Exam #:

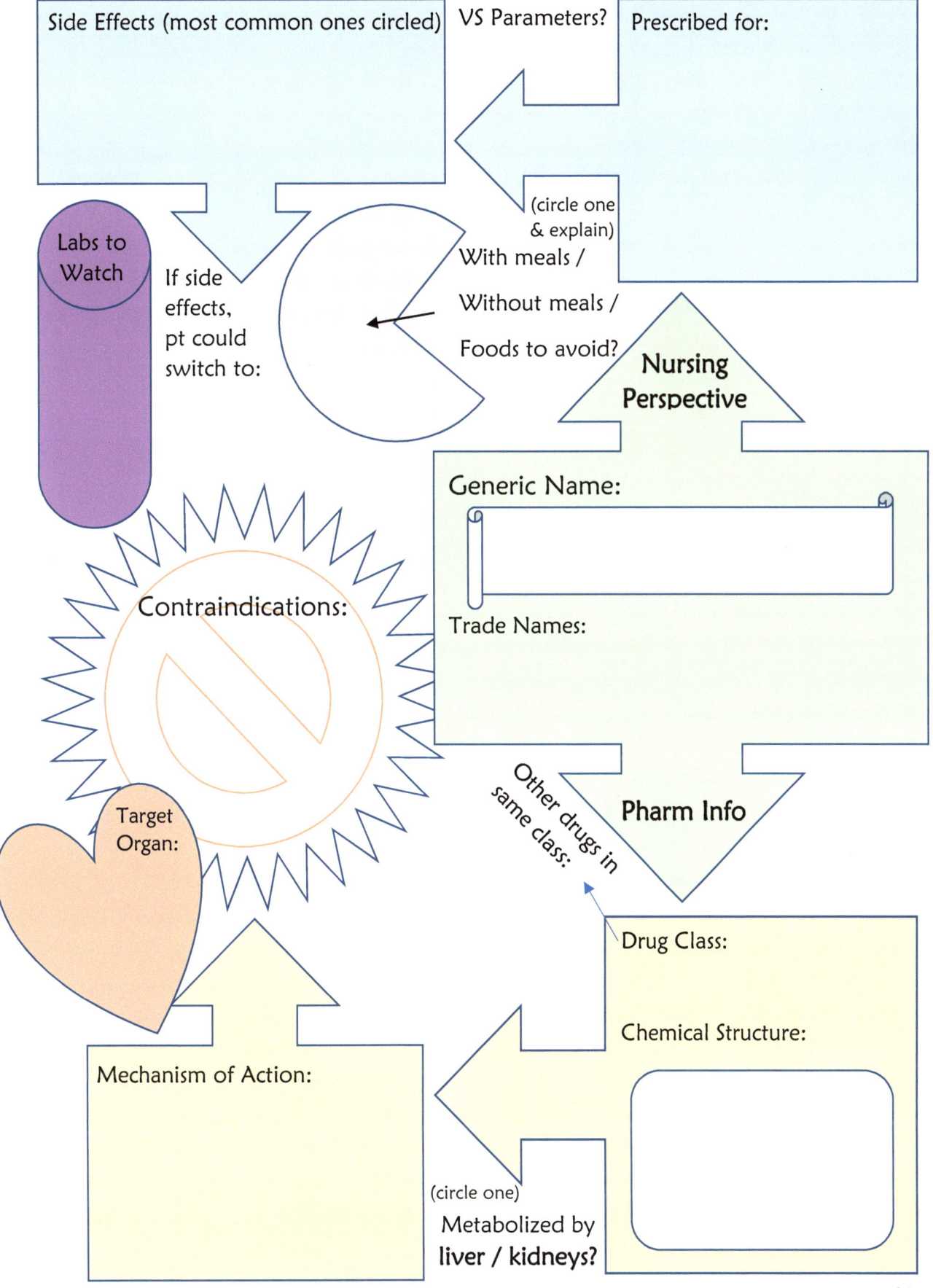

Date: Class: This content will appear on Exam #:

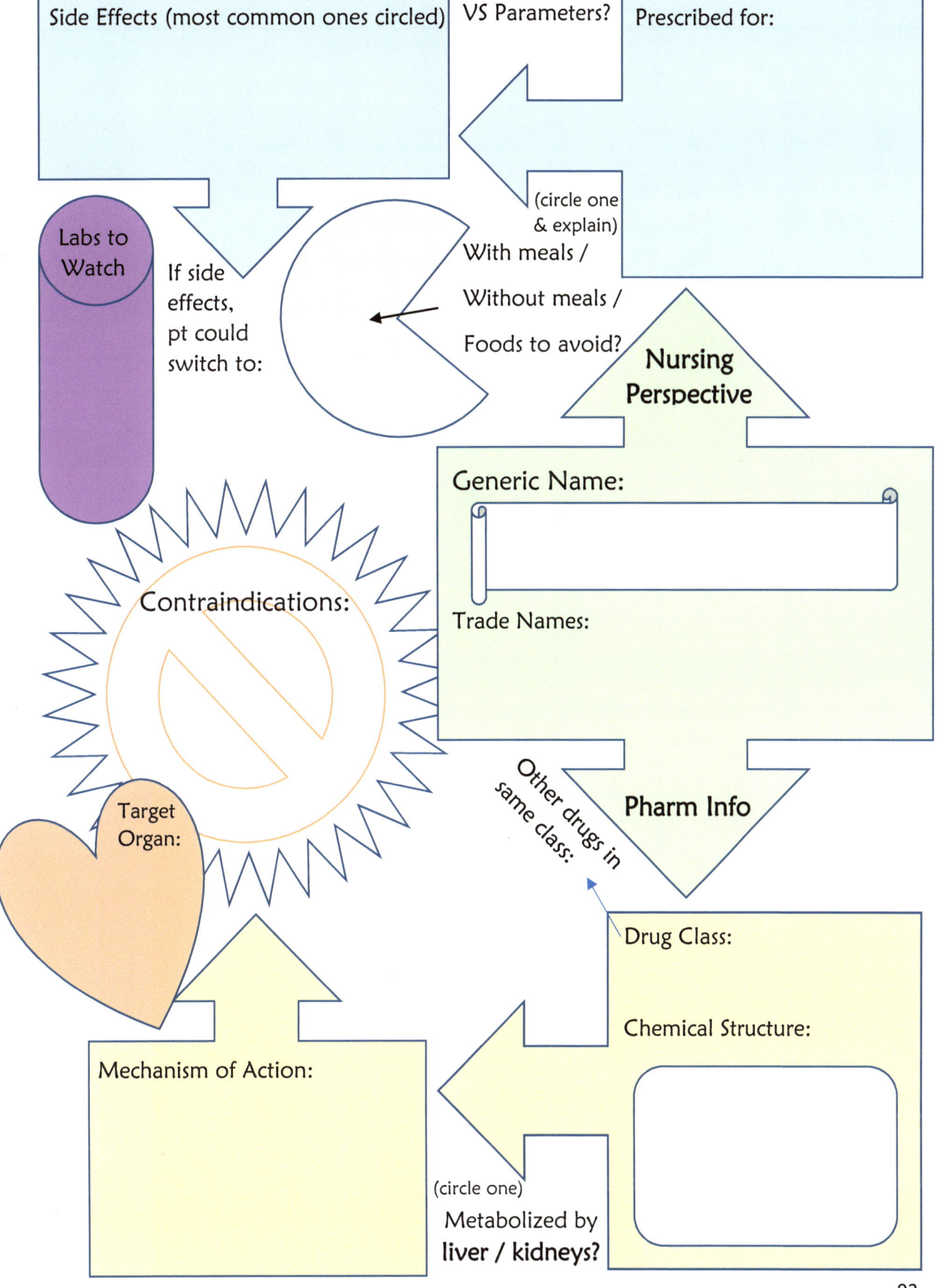

Date: Class: This content will appear on Exam #:

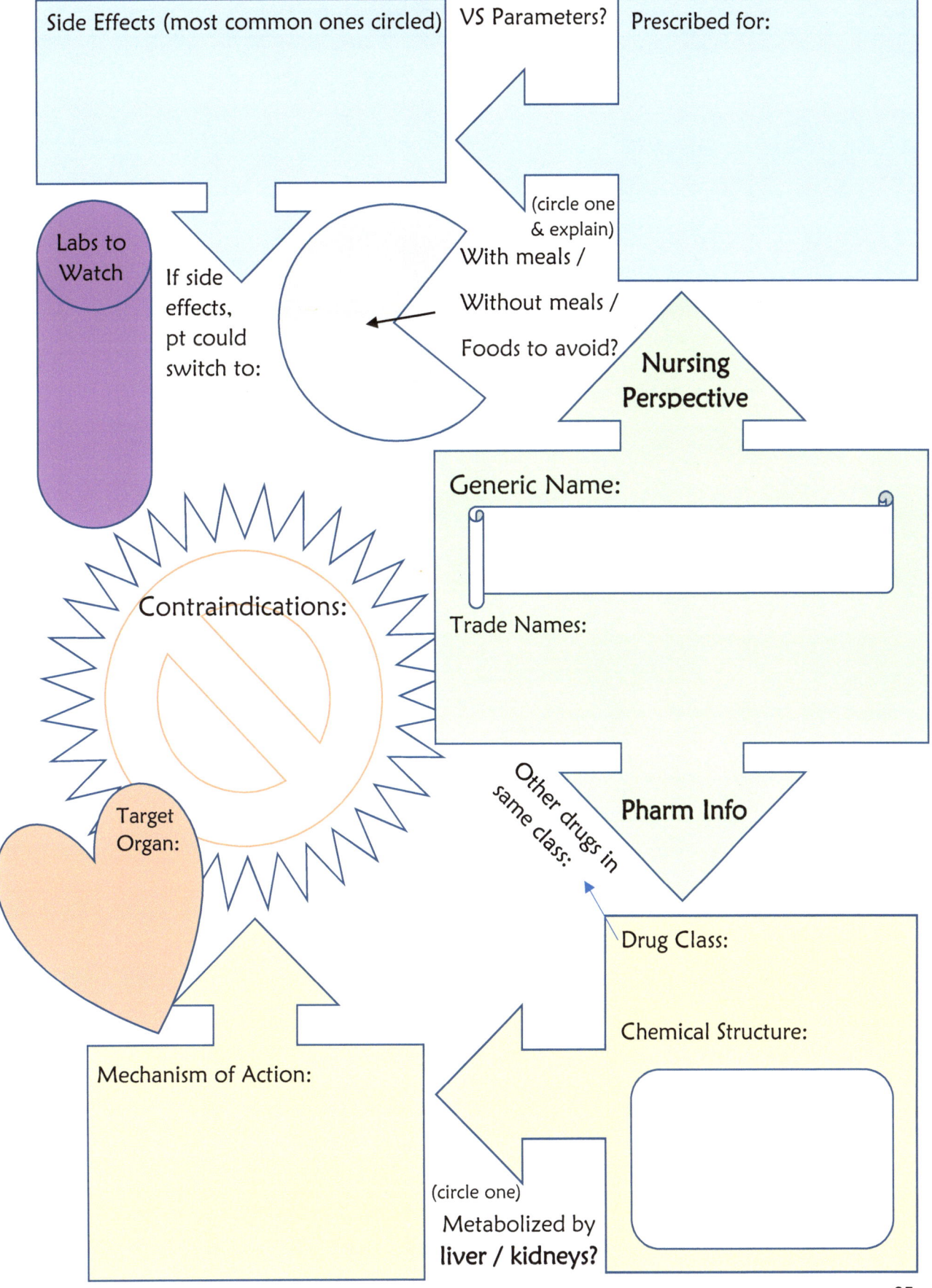

Date: Class: This content will appear on Exam #:

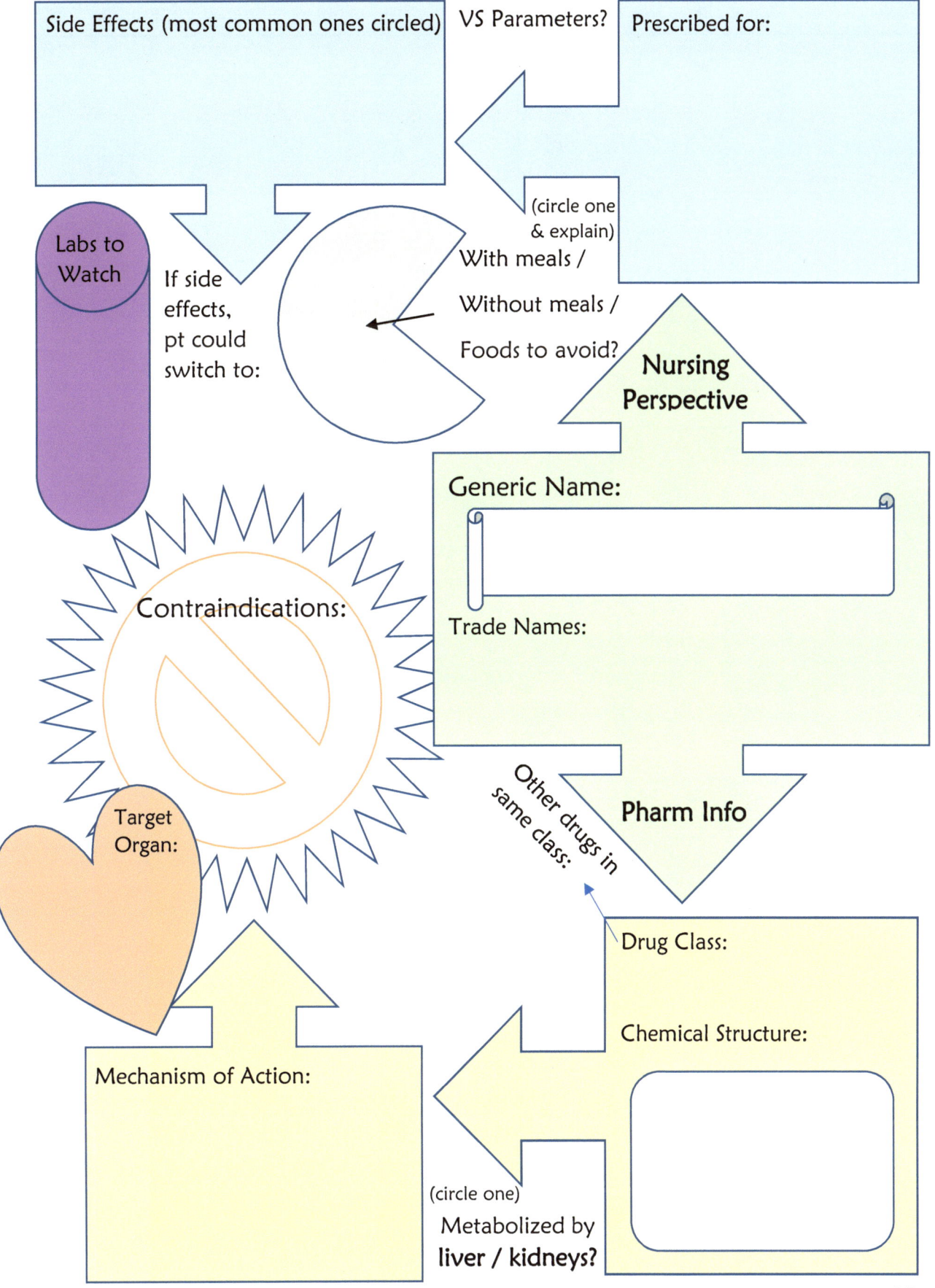

Date: Class: This content will appear on Exam #:

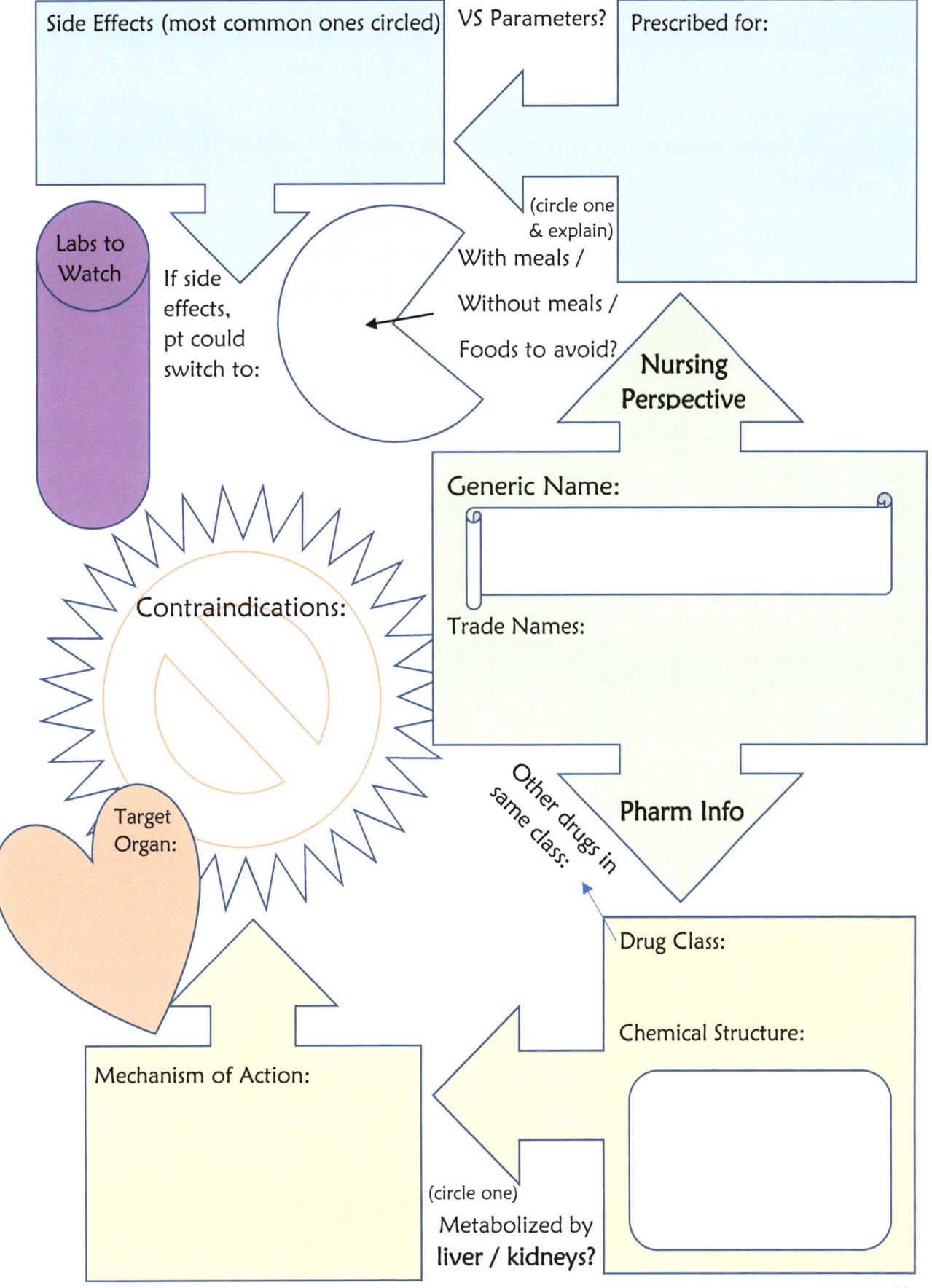